C000114941

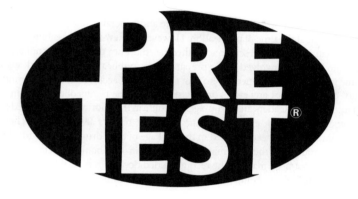

# Pharmacology
## PreTest® Self-Assessment and Review

# NOTICE

Medicine is an ever-changing science. As new research and clinical experience broaden our knowledge, changes in treatment and drug therapy are required. The author and the publisher of this work have checked with sources believed to be reliable in their efforts to provide information that is complete and generally in accord with the standards accepted at the time of publication. However, in view of the possibility of human error or changes in medical sciences, neither the editor nor the publisher nor any other party who has been involved in the preparation or publication of this work warrants that the information contained herein is in every respect accurate or complete and they are not responsible for any errors or omissions or for the results obtained from use of such information. Readers are encouraged to confirm the information contained herein with other sources. For example and in particular, readers are advised to check the product information sheet included in the package of each drug they plan to administer to be certain that the information contained in this book is accurate and that changes have not been made in the recommended dose or in the contraindications for administration. This recommendation is of particular importance in connection with new or infrequently used drugs.

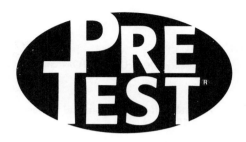

# Pharmacology
## PreTest® Self-Assessment and Review
### Ninth Edition

EDITOR
**ARNOLD STERN, M.D., PH.D.**
Professor of Pharmacology
New York University Medical Center
New York, New York

STUDENT REVIEWERS
**Daniel S. Gabbay**
SUNY School of Medicine
at Stony Brook
Stony Brook, NY

**Jodi Rosenbleet**
Temple University School of Medicine
Philadelphia, PA

 **McGraw-Hill**
**Health Professions Division**
**PreTest® Series**

NEW YORK   ST. LOUIS   SAN FRANCISCO   AUCKLAND
BOGOTÁ   CARACAS   LISBON   LONDON   MADRID
MEXICO CITY   MILAN   MONTREAL   NEW DELHI
SAN JUAN   SINGAPORE   SYDNEY   TOKYO   TORONTO

# Mcgraw-Hill

A Division of The **McGraw·Hill** Companies

**Pharmacology: PreTest® Self-Assessment and Review, Ninth Edition International Editions 1999**

Exclusive rights by McGraw-Hill Book Co-Singapore, for manufacture and export. This book cannot be re-exported from the country to which it is consigned by McGraw-Hill.

2 3 4 5 6 7 8 9 0 KKP PMP 2 0 9 9

**ISBN 0-07-052694-X**

*The editors were John J. Dolan, Susan R. Noujaim, and Peter McCurdy. The production supervisor was Helene G. Landers. The text designer was Jim Sullivan/RepoCat Graphics & Editorial Services. The cover designer was Li Chen Chang/Pinpoint. This book was set in Berkeley by V & M Graphics.*

**When ordering this title, use ISBN 0-07-116685-8**

Printed in Singapore

# CONTENTS

# PREFACE

In this ninth edition of *Pharmacology: PreTest® Self-Assessment and Review*, significant changes and improvements have been made. Questions that use clinical vignettes have been added; the responses require interpretation and data synthesis. The number of items per group of matching questions has been reduced in accordance with the new format used on United States Medical Licensing Examination (USMLE), Step 1. A High-Yield Facts section containing two sample Drug Classification Tables has been added; these tables serve as simple examples for collating and comparing information about various drug classes. References have been updated, and this section is preceded by a List of Abbreviations and Acronyms used throughout the book.

The author remains indebted to his students and colleagues at New York University Medical Center for their continuing support and encouragement.

# INTRODUCTION

Each *PreTest® Self-Assessment and Review* allows medical students to comprehensively and conveniently assess and review their knowledge of a particular basic science—in this instance, Pharmacology. The 485 questions parallel the format and degree of difficulty of the questions found in the United States Medical Licensing Examination (USMLE) Step 1. Practicing physicians who want to hone their skills before USMLE Step 3 or recertification may find this to be a good beginning in their review process.

Each question is accompanied by an answer, a paragraph explanation, and a specific page reference to an appropriate textbook. A bibliography listing sources can be found following the last chapter of this text.

Before each chapter, a list of key terms or classifications of drugs or both is included to aid review. In addition, suggestions for effective study and review have been added below.

The most effective method of using this book is to complete one chapter at a time. Prepare yourself for each chapter by reviewing from your notes and favorite text the drugs listed at the beginning of each section. You should concentrate especially on the prototype drugs, which are marked by an asterisk. Then proceed to indicate your answer by each question, allowing yourself not more than one minute for each question. In this way you will be approximating the time limits imposed by the Step.

After you finish going through the questions in the section, spend as much time as you need verifying your answers and carefully reading the explanations provided. Pay special attention to the explanations for the questions you answered incorrectly—but read *every* explanation. The editors of this material have designed the explanations to reinforce and supplement the information tested by the questions. If you feel you need further information about the material covered, consult and study the references indicated.

# SUGGESTIONS FOR EFFECTIVE STUDY AND REVIEW

The study of pharmacology is not different from that of the other basic medical sciences. For most students, pharmacology may seem more relevant than other subjects to the practice of clinical medicine. It has the advantage of coming last in the curriculum of basic sciences. Nevertheless, the disadvantage of pharmacology is the need to commit to memory an enormous number of names and facts about numerous drugs and furthermore to relate these to each other and to clinical medicine. Most students find it advantageous to learn a classification of drugs that enables them to immediately place a drug into a category that characterizes the likely pharmacology. In addition, the main or original drug in each category (the prototype drug) should be thoroughly studied. The close relatives need merely to be known by name and with reference to their advantages over the prototype drug.

Although it may be obvious, it is still worth repeating that a minimum knowledge of prototype drugs consists of the following:

1.  *Chemistry.* You should be able to recognize the structural formula. Are there any structure-activity relationships (SARs)? What is the main ring structure? steroid? quinoline? benzodiazepine? sympathetic amine? etc.

2.  *Mechanism of Action.* This usually consists of two parts: (1) molecular and (2) cellular or physiologic. Mechanisms of action mainly explain the pharmacodynamics or effects on organ systems that are of most use in a clinical knowledge of the drug. For example, does the drug lower blood pressure? if so, does it do so by vasodilation, negative inotropic effects on the heart, central nervous system mechanisms? etc.

3.  *Pharmacokinetics.* This covers absorption, distribution, and elimination of the drug. What is the usual route of administration of the drug? What is its half-life? degree of protein binding? etc. The dose of the drug is usually not asked in modern examinations. However, the means by which dosage can increase or decrease blood levels of drugs must be known. This is the essence of pharmacokinetics. Concepts and formulas for determining half-life, volume of distribution, and clearance must be understood and memorized. They are listed at the beginning of the first chapter, General Principles.

4.  *Clinical Use.* You should know Food and Drug Administration (FDA) indications plus medically accepted uses.

5. *Toxicity.* This includes adverse reactions and serious toxicities, such as nephritis, hepatitis, blood dyscrasia, etc. You should know important drug interactions.

With respect to names of drugs, the generic name must be known even though the trade name is often more commonly used. In this text, the generic name is always used. It is advantageous to memorize certain endings because they give a clue as to the category in which a drug belongs; there are many exceptions, but these endings do help memory. The following are examples of endings of generic names:

| Suffix | Drug Class | Examples |
|---|---|---|
| -ane | volatile general anesthetics | halothane, enflurane |
| -azepam | antianxiety drugs | diazepam, lorazepam |
| -azine | phenothiazine-like antipsychotic drugs | chlorpromazine, thioridazine |
| -bital | barbiturate sedative hypnotic drugs | secobarbital |
| -caine | local anesthetics | cocaine, procaine |
| -cillin | penicillins | nafcillin, piperacillin |
| -cycline | tetracycline-type antibiotics | doxycycline, methacycline |
| -mycin | aminoglycoside antibiotics | streptomycin, kanamycin |
| -olol | (-adrenergic blockers | propranolol, metoprolol |
| -opril | angiotensin-converting enzyme inhibitors | captopril, enalapril |
| -statin | HMG-CoA (3-hydroxy-3-methylglutaryl-coenzyme A) reductase inhibitors | lovastatin, pravastatin |
| -zosin | postsynaptic $\alpha$-receptor blockers | terazosin, prazosin |

# GENERAL PRINCIPLES

Drug-receptor interaction
Dose-response relationship
  Graded dose-response curve
  Quantal dose-response curve
  Time-action curves
  Therapeutic index
  Drug assays, biologic versus
    chemical
Receptors
  Nature of the drug-receptor
    interaction
  Structure and activity relation-
    ship (SAR)
  Physical chemistry of the
    drug-receptor association
  Relationship to Michaelis-
    Menten enzyme kinetics
  Simultaneous action of two drugs
  Additive effects
  Potentiation
  Synergism
  Competitive antagonism
  Noncompetitive antagonism
  Other factors in drug-receptor
    interaction
  Tolerance
  Tachyphylaxis
  Up and down regulation by
    the number of receptors
  Scatchard plot
Molecular Models of Receptors
  and Transduction Mechanisms
1. Ion channel receptors
  Nicotine

$\gamma$-aminobutyric acid (GABA)
Glycine
Glutamate ($N$-methyl-D-
  aspartate antagonists
  [NMDA] quisqualate, kainate)
Transduction mechanism =
  ionic
2. Receptor-G protein–effector
  system
$\beta$-adrenergic
Muscarinic
Serotonin
Angiotensin
Rhodopsin
Transduction mechanism = G
  protein linked by guanine
  diphosphate and triphos-
  phate (GDP-GTP) linked to
  adenylate-cyclase activity,
  phospholipase, potassium
  (K), and calcium (Ca) channels
3. Receptor tyrosine kinases
  Erythrocyte growth factor (EGF)
  Platelet-derived growth factor
  (PDGF)
  Insulin
  Transduction mechanism =
    Activation of protein kinases
4. Steroid hormone receptors
  Thyroid hormone
  Vitamin D
  Estrogen
  Progesterone
  Glucocorticoid

First order

$$\text{Slope} = \frac{-k}{2.303}$$

Half-life $(t^{1}/_{2})$

$$t^{1}/_{2} = \frac{0.693}{k}$$

Zero-order rate equation
Volume of distribution $(V_d)$

$$V_d = \frac{\text{Total amount of drug in the body}}{\text{concentration of drug in plasma}}$$

Distribution phase vs elimination phase determined as plasma concentration $\times$ time curves
Clearance

$$CL_{total} = V_d \times k_e = \frac{0.693 \times V_d}{t^{1}/_{2}}$$

$$t^{1}/_{2} = \frac{0.693 \times V_d}{CL_{total}}$$

Dosage regimens and pharmacokinetic profiles
Single doses
IV
Oral
Bioavailability
Multiple doses
Interval between doses and accumulation
Continuous IV infusion
Multiple oral dosing
Clinical Pharmacology
Definition and scope
Statistical and epidemiologic approaches
Bioavailability and bioequivalence
Placebo effect
Drug Interactions
Mechanisms
Enzyme stimulation (induction)
Enzyme inhibition
Gastrointestinal (GI) absorption changes
Protein binding
Adrenergic mechanisms
Cholinergic mechanisms
Neuromuscular junction
Drug biotransformation
Renal tubular transport
Urinary pH and drug excretion
Factors Affecting Drug Dosage
Age, sex, and weight
Pregnancy and lactation
Renal disease
Hepatic disease
Pharmacogenetics
Development of New Drugs
Animal vs human doses
Single-dose methodology
Open studies
Blind and double-blind studies
Regulation by the Food and Drug Administration
Investigational new drug (IND)
New drug application (NDA)
Phase I, II, III, and IV studies
Postmarketing surveillance
Ethics of Human Investigation
Institutional Review Board (IRB)
Fate of marketed drugs

*Scatter diagram*

# Questions

**DIRECTIONS:** Each question below contains several suggested responses. Select the **one best** response to each question.

1. Of the many types of plots of data that are used to help explain the pharmacodynamics of drugs, which plot is very useful for determining the total number of receptors and the affinity of a drug for those receptors in a tissue or membrane?

a. graded dose-response curve
b. quantal dose-response curve
c. scatchard plot
d. double-reciprocal plot
e. Michaelis-Menten plot

2. Which route of administration is most likely to subject a drug to a first-pass effect?

a. IV
b. inhalational
c. oral
d. sublingual (SL)
e. IM

3. Two drugs may act on the same tissue or organ through independent receptors, resulting in effects in opposite directions. This is known as

a. physiologic antagonism
b. chemical antagonism
c. competitive antagonism
d. irreversible antagonism
e. dispositional antagonism

## Questions 4–7

A new aminoglycoside antibiotic (5 mg/kg) was infused IV over 30 min to a 70-kg volunteer. The plasma concentrations of the drug were measured at various times after the end of the infusion, as recorded in the table and shown in the figure below.

| Time After Dosing Stopped (h) | Plasma Aminoglycoside Concentration (μg/mL) |
|:---:|:---:|
| 0.0 | 18.0 |
| 0.5 | 10.0 |
| 1.0 | 5.8 |
| 2.0 | 4.6 |
| 3.0 | 3.7 |
| 4.0 | 3.0 |
| 5.0 | 2.4 |
| 6.0 | 1.9 |
| 8.0 | 1.3 |

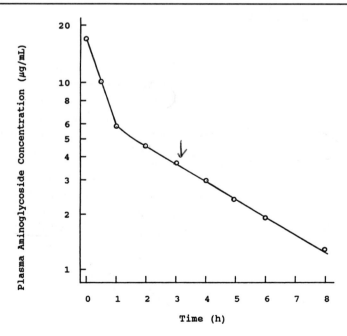

$t\frac{1}{2} \times 4 \rightarrow$ (elimination of the Drug)

**4.** The elimination half-life ($t_{1/2}$) of the aminoglycoside in this patient was approximately

a.   0.6 h
b.   1.2 h
c.   2.1 h
d.   3.1 h
e.   4.2 h

**5.** The elimination rate constant ($k_e$) of the aminoglycoside in this patient was approximately

a.   0.15 h$^{-1}$        $Ke = 0.693$
b.   0.22 h$^{-1}$              $\overline{t\frac{1}{2}}$
c.   0.33 h$^{-1}$
d.   0.60 h$^{-1}$
e.   1.13 h$^{-1}$

**6.** The apparent volume of distribution ($V_d$) of the drug in this patient was approximately

a.   0.62 L
b.   19 L
c.   50 L
d.   110 L
e.   350 L

**7.** The total body clearance ($CL_{total}$) of the drug in this patient was approximately

a.   11 L/h
b.   23 L/h
c.   35 L/h
d.   47 L/h
e.   65 L/h

**8.** If a drug is repeatedly administered at dosing intervals equal to its elimination half-life, the number of doses required for the plasma concentration of the drug to reach the steady state is

a.   2 to 3
b.   4 to 5
c.   6 to 7
d.   8 to 9
e.   10 or more

**9.** The pharmacokinetic value that most reliably reflects the amount of drug reaching the target tissue after oral administration is the

a.   peak blood concentration
b.   time to peak blood concentration
c.   product of the $V_d$ and the first-order rate constant
d.   $V_d$
e.   area under the blood concentration-time curve (AUC)

**10.** It was determined that 95% of an oral 80-mg dose of verapamil was absorbed in a 70-kg test subject. However, because of extensive biotransformation during its first pass through the portal circulation, the bioavailability of verapamil was only 25%. Assuming a liver blood flow of 1500 mL/min, the hepatic clearance of verapamil in this situation was

a.   60 mL/min
b.   375 mL/min
c.   740 mL/min
d.   1110 mL/min
e.   1425 mL/min

**11.** Drug products have many types of names. Of the following types of names that are applied to drugs, the one that is the official name and refers only to that drug and not to a particular product is the

a. generic name    *Salbutamol*
b. trade name    *Ventolin*
c. brand name
d. chemical name
e. proprietary name

(4)

**12.** Which of the following is classified as belonging to the tyrosine kinase family of receptors?

a. GABA$_A$ receptor
b. β-adrenergic receptor
c. insulin receptor
d. nicotinic-II receptor
e. hydrocortisone receptor

**13.** Identical doses of a capsule preparation (X) and a tablet preparation (Y) of the same drug were compared on a blood concentration-time plot with respect to peak concentration, time to peak concentration, and AUC after oral administration as shown in the figure below. This comparison was made to determine which of the following?

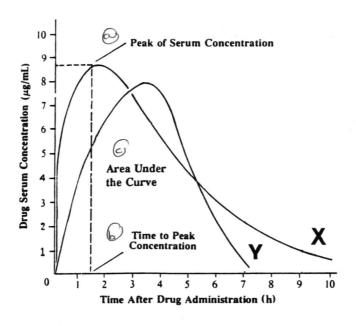

a. potency
b. extent of plasma protein binding
c. bioequivalence
d. therapeutic effectiveness
e. none of the above

**DIRECTIONS:** Each numbered question or incomplete statement below is NEGATIVELY phrased. Select the **one best** lettered response.

**14.** All the following characteristics are associated with the process of facilitated diffusion of drugs EXCEPT

a. the transport mechanism becomes saturated at high drug concentrations

b. the process is selective for certain ionic or structural configurations of the drug

c. if two compounds are transported by the same mechanism, one will competitively inhibit the transport of the other

d. the drug crosses the membrane against a concentration gradient and the process requires cellular energy

e. the transport process can be inhibited noncompetitively by substances that interfere with cellular metabolism

**15.** The route of excretion for drugs or their metabolic derivatives that is quantitatively the LEAST significant is which of the following?

a. biliary tract
b. kidneys
c. lungs
d. feces
e. milk

**16.** All the following are phase I biotransformation reactions EXCEPT

a. sulfoxide formation
b. nitro reduction
c. ester hydrolysis
d. sulfate conjugation   / G lucuronide
e. deamination

**17.** An enteric-coated dosage form can be used to avoid all the following problems possible from oral drug administration EXCEPT

a. irritation to the gastric mucosa with nausea and vomiting

b. destruction of the drug by gastric acid or digestive enzymes

c. unpleasant taste of the drug

d. formation of nonabsorbable drug-food complexes

e. variability in absorption caused by fluctuations in gastric emptying time

**18.** All the following statements concerning receptors bound to plasma membranes, their interaction with ligands, and the biologic response to this interaction are true EXCEPT

a. structurally, these receptors have hydrophobic amino acid domains, which are in contact with the membrane, and hydrophilic regions, which extend into the extracellular fluid and the cytoplasm

b. chemical interactions of ligands with these receptors may involve the formation of many types of bonds, including ionic, hydrogen, Van der Waals, and covalent

c. ligand-receptor interactions are often stereospecific, i.e., one stereoisomer is usually more potent than the other

d. a ligand that acts as an agonist at membrane-bound receptors increases the activity of an intracellular second messenger

e. activation of membrane-bound receptors and subsequent intracellular events elicit a biologic response through the transcription of DNA

**19.** All the following statements concerning binding of drugs to plasma proteins are true EXCEPT

a. acidic drugs generally bind to plasma albumin; basic drugs preferentially bind to $\alpha_1$-acidic glycoprotein

b. plasma protein binding is a reversible process

c. binding sites on plasma proteins are nonselective and drugs with similar physicochemical characteristics compete for these limited sites

d. the fraction of the drug in the plasma that is bound is inactive and generally unavailable for systemic distribution

e. plasma protein binding generally limits renal tubular secretion and biotransformation

**20.** All the following statements concerning drug distribution into and out of the central nervous system (CNS) are true EXCEPT

a. the blood-brain barrier, which involves drug movement through glial cell membranes as well as capillary membranes, is the main hindrance to drug distribution to the CNS
b. most drugs enter the CNS by simple diffusion at rates proportional to the lipid solubility of the nonionized form of the drug
c. receptor-mediated transport allows certain peptides to gain access to the brain
d. strongly ionized drugs freely enter the CNS through carrier-mediated transport systems
e. some drugs leave the CNS by passing from the cerebrospinal fluid into the dural blood sinuses through the arachnoid villi

**21.** The greater proportion of the dose of a drug administered orally will be absorbed in the small intestine. However, on the assumption that passive transport of the nonionized form of a drug determines its rate of absorption, which of the following compounds will be absorbed to the LEAST extent in the stomach?

a. ampicillin ($pK_a = 2.5$)
b. aspirin ($pK_a = 3.0$)
c. warfarin ($pK_a = 5.0$)
d. phenobarbital ($pK_a = 7.4$)
e. propranolol ($pK_a = 9.4$)

**DIRECTIONS:** Each group of questions below consists of lettered headings followed by a set of numbered items. For each numbered item select the **one** lettered heading with which it is **most** closely associated. Each lettered heading may be used **once, more than once, or not at all.**

**Questions 22–24**

For each type of drug interaction below, select the pair of substances that illustrates it with a REDUCTION in drug effectiveness:

a. tetracycline and milk
b. amobarbital and secobarbital
c. isoproterenol and propranolol
d. soap and benzalkonium chloride
e. sulfamethoxazole and trimethoprim

c **22.** Therapeutic interaction
$\beta \longrightarrow \beta$ Blocker

d **23.** Physical interaction

a **24.** Chemical interaction
$( TC \longrightarrow milk )$

**Questions 25–27**

For each description of a drug response below, choose the term with which it is most likely to be associated:

a. supersensitivity
b. tachyphylaxis
c. tolerance
d. hyposensitivity
e. anaphylaxis

e **25.** Immunologically mediated reaction to drug observed soon after administration
*Anaphylaxis*

b **26.** A rapid reduction in the effect of a given dose of a drug after only one or two doses
*Tachyphylaxis*

a **27.** Hyperreactivity to a drug seen as a result of denervation
*Supersensitivity*

## Questions 28–30

For each component of a time-action curve listed below, choose the lettered interval (shown on the diagram) with which it is most closely associated:

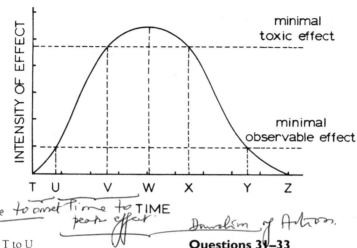

*time to onset* *time to*
*peak effect* **TIME**    *Duration of Action.*

a.  T to U
b.  T to V
c.  T to W
d.  T to Z
e.  U to V
f.  U to W
g.  U to X
h.  U to Y
i.  V to X
j.  X to Y

*C* **28.** Time to peak effect

*a* **29.** Time to onset of action

*l* **30.** Duration of action

## Questions 31–33

For each description below, select the transmembranal transport mechanism it best defines:

a.  filtration
b.  simple diffusion
c.  facilitated diffusion
d.  active transport
e.  endocytosis

*Simple diffusion*

*b* **31.** Lipid-soluble drugs cross the membrane at a rate proportional to the concentration gradient across the membrane and the lipid:water partition coefficient of the drug *filtration*

**a** **32.** Bulk flow of water through membrane pores, resulting from osmotic differences across the membrane, transports drug molecules that fit through the membrane pores

*active transport*

**d** **33.** After binding to a proteinaceous membrane carrier, drugs are carried across the membrane (with the expenditure of cellular energy), where they are released

*Cyt P450*

**g** **34.** A group of iron (Fe)-containing isoenzymes that activate molecular oxygen to a form capable of interacting with organic substrates

**a**

**35.** The component that provides reducing equivalents for the enzyme system   NADPH

**d**

**36.** A flavoprotein that accepts reducing equivalents and transfers them to the catalytic enzyme

NADPH — Cyt P450

## Questions 34–36

Lipid-soluble xenobiotics are commonly biotransformed by oxidation in the drug-metabolizing microsomal system (DMMS). For each description below, choose the component of the microsomal mixed-function oxidase system with which it is most closely associated:

a.  nicotinamide adenine dinucleotide phosphate (NADPH)
b.  cytochrome *a*
c.  adenosine triphosphate (ATP)
d.  NADPH–cytochrome P-450 reductase
e.  monoamine oxidase (MAO)
f.  cyclooxygenase
g.  cytochrome P-450

# GENERAL PRINCIPLES

## Answers

**1. The answer is c.** (*DiPalma, 4/e, pp 22–23. Hardman and Limbird, 9/e, pp 37–38.*) Based on the concept that, for most situations, the association of a drug with its receptor is reversible, the following reaction applies:

$$D + R \underset{k_2}{\overset{k_1}{\rightleftharpoons}} DR \rightarrow Effect$$

where D is the concentration of free drug, R is the concentration of receptors, DR is the concentration of drug bound to its receptors, and $K_D$ (equal to $k_2/k_1$) is the equilibrium dissociation constant. The affinity of a drug for its receptor is estimated from the dissociation constant in that its reciprocal, $1/K_D$, is the affinity constant. All the plots listed in the question can be used to quantitate some aspect of drug action. For example, $K_D$ can be determined from the Michaelis-Menten relationship, graded dose-response curves, and the Scatchard plot. However, only the Scatchard plot can be used to determine the total number of receptors in a tissue or membrane. This is accomplished by measuring the binding of a radioactively labeled drug to a membrane or tissue preparation in vitro. A Scatchard plot of the binding of $^3$H-yohimbine to $\alpha_2$-adrenergic receptors on human platelet membranes is shown on the following page as an example. A plot of DR/D (bound/free drug) versus DR (bound drug) yields a slope of $1/K_D$ (the affinity constant) and an x intercept of R (total number of receptors).

This type of analysis is very useful in certain therapeutic situations. For example, Scatchard analysis is used to determine the number of estrogen receptors present in a biopsy of breast tissue prior to developing a drug treatment regimen for breast cancer in a patient.

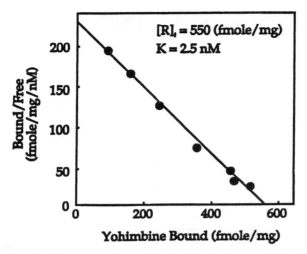

**Yohimbine Bound (fmole/mg)**

(From Neubig RR, Gantros RD, and Brasier RS: *Mol Pharmacol* 28:475–486, 1985, with permission.)


**2. The answer is c.** *(DiPalma, 4/e, pp 48–49, 61–62. Hardman and Limbird, 9/e, p 5.)* The first-pass effect is commonly considered to involve the biotransformation of a drug during its first passage through the portal circulation of the liver. Drugs that are administered orally and rectally enter the portal circulation of the liver and can be biotransformed by this organ prior to reaching the systemic circulation. Therefore, drugs with a *high* first-pass effect are highly biotransformed quickly, which reduces the oral bioavailability and the systemic blood concentrations of the compounds. Administration by the IV, IM, and SL routes allows the drug to attain concentrations in the systemic circulation and to be distributed throughout the body prior to hepatic metabolism. In most cases, drugs administered by inhalation are not subjected to a significant first-pass effect unless the respiratory tissue is a major site for the drug's biotransformation.


**3. The answer is a.** *(DiPalma, 4/e, p 24. Hardman and Limbird, 9/e, p 68.)* Physiologic, or *functional, antagonism* occurs when two drugs produce opposite effects on the same physiologic function, often by interacting with different types of receptors. A practical example of this is the use of epinephrine as a bronchodilator to counteract the bronchoconstriction that occurs following histamine release from mast cells in the respiratory tract during a severe allergic reaction. Histamine constricts the bronchioles by stimulating histamine $H_1$ receptors in the tissue; epinephrine relaxes this tissue through its agonistic activity on $\beta_2$-adrenergic receptors. *Chemical antagonism* results when two drugs combine with each other chemically and the activity of one or both is blocked. For example, dimercaprol chelates lead and reduces the toxicity of this heavy metal. *Competitive antagonism*, or *inactivation*, occurs when two compounds compete for the same receptor site; this is a reversible interaction. Thus, atropine blocks the effects of acetylcholine on the heart by competing with the neurotransmitter for binding to cardiac muscarinic receptors. *Irreversible antagonism* generally results from the binding of an antagonist to the same receptor site as the agonist by covalent interaction or by a very slowly dissociating noncovalent interaction. An example of this antagonism is the blockade produced by phenoxybenzamine on $\alpha$-adrenergic receptors, resulting in a long-lasting reduction in the activity of norepinephrine. *Dispositional antagonism* occurs when one drug alters the pharmacokinetics (absorption, distribution, biotransformation, or excretion) of a second drug so that less of the active compound reaches the target tissue. For example, phenobarbital induces the biotransformation of warfarin, reducing its anticoagulant activity.

**4. The answer is d.** *(DiPalma, 4/e, pp 55–58. Katzung, 7/e, pp 35–40.)* The figure that accompanies the question shows an elimination pattern with two distinct components, which typifies a two-compartment model. The upper portion of the line represents the $\alpha$ phase, which is the distribution of the drug from the tissues that receive high rates of blood flow (the central compartment, e.g., the brain, heart, kidney, and lungs) to the tissues with lower rates of blood flow (the peripheral compartment, e.g., skeletal muscle, adipose tissue, and bone). Once distribution to all tissue is complete, equilibrium occurs throughout the body. The elimination of the drug from the body (the $\beta$ phase) is represented by the lower linear portion of the line; this part of the line is used to determine the elimination half-life of the drug. At 2 h after dosing, the plasma concentration was 4.6 µg/mL; at 5 h the concentration was 2.4 µg/mL. Therefore the plasma concentration of this aminoglycoside decreased to one-half in approximately 3 h—its half-life. In addition, drug elimination usually occurs according to first-order kinetics, i.e., a linear relationship is obtained when the drug concentration is plotted on a logarithmic scale versus time on an arithmetic scale (a semilogarithmic plot).

**5. The answer is b.** *(DiPalma, 4/e, pp 57–58. Katzung, 7/e, p 39.)* The fraction change in drug concentration per unit of time for any first-order process is expressed by $k_e$. This constant is related to the half-life $(t_{1/2})$ by the equation $k_e t_{1/2} = 0.693$. The units of $k_e$ are time$^{-1}$, while the $t_{1/2}$ is expressed in units of time. By substitution of the appropriate value for half-life estimated from the data from the graph or table accompanying the question (the $\beta$ phase) into the above equation, rearranged to solve for $k_e$, the answer is calculated as follows:

$$k_e = \frac{0.693}{t_{1/2}} = \frac{0.693}{3.0 \text{ h}} = 0.23 \text{ h}^{-1}$$

The problem can also be solved mathematically:

$$\log[A] = \log[A_o] - \frac{k_e}{2.303} t$$

where $[A_o]$ is the initial drug concentration, $[A]$ is the final drug concentration, t is the time interval between the two values, and $k_e$ is the elimination rate constant. For example, by solving for $k_e$ using the plasma concentration values at 2 and 5 h,

$$\log[2.4 \text{ μg/mL}] = \log[4.6 \text{ μg/mL}] - \frac{k_e}{2.303} 3 \text{ h}$$

$k_e$ will equal 0.22 h$^{-1}$.

**6. The answer is c.** *(DiPalma, 4/e, pp 58–60. Katzung, 7/e, p 34.)* The apparent $V_d$ is defined as the volume of fluid into which a drug appears to distribute with a concentration equal to that of plasma, or the volume of fluid necessary to dissolve the drug and yield the same concentration as that found in plasma. By convention, the value of the plasma concentration at zero time is used. In this problem, a hypothetical plasma concentration of the drug at zero time (7 μg/mL) can be estimated by extrapolating the linear portion of the elimination curve (the $\beta$ phase) back to zero time. Therefore, the apparent $V_d$ is calculated by

$$V_d = \frac{\text{Total amount of drug in the body}}{\text{Drug concentration in plasma at zero time}}$$

Since the total amount of drug in the body is the IV dose, 350 mg, i.e., 5 mg/kg × 70 kg, and the estimated plasma concentration at zero time is 7 μg/mL, substitution of these numbers in the equation yields the apparent $V_d$:

$$V_d = \frac{350 \text{ mg}}{7 \text{ μg/mL}} = 50 \text{ L}$$

**7. The answer is a.** *(DiPalma, 4/e, p 60. Katzung, 6/e, pp 35, 39.)* Clearance by an organ is defined as the apparent volume of a biologic fluid from which a drug is removed by elimination processes per unit of time. The total body clearance ($CL_{total}$) is defined as the sum of clearances of all the organs and tissues that eliminate a drug. $CL_{total}$ is influenced by the apparent $V_d$ and $k_e$. The more rapidly a drug is cleared, the greater is the value of $CL_{total}$. Therefore, for the new aminoglycoside in this patient,

$$CL_{total} = V_d k_e = (50 \text{ L}) (0.22 \text{ h}^{-1}) = 11 \text{ L/h}$$

**8. The answer is b.** *(DiPalma, 4/e, pp 62–63. Hardman and Limbird, 9/e, p 23.)* When a drug is administered in multiple doses and each dose is given prior to the complete elimination of the previous dose, the mean plasma concentration (C) of the drug during each dose interval rises as shown in the following figure:

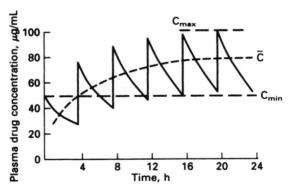

(From DiPalma and DiGregorio, with permission.)

The plasma concentration will continue to rise until it reaches a plateau, or steady state. At this time, the plasma concentration will fluctuate between a maximum ($C_{max}$) and a minimum ($C_{min}$) level, but more importantly, the amount of drug eliminated per dose interval will equal the amount of drug absorbed per dose. When a drug is given at a dosing interval equal to its elimination half-life, it will reach 50% of its steady state plasma concentration after one half-life, 75% after two half-lives, 87.5% after three, 93.75% after four, and 96.87% after five. Thus, from a practical viewpoint, regardless of the magnitude of the dose or the half-life, the steady state will be achieved in four to five half-lives.

**9. The answer is e.** (*DiPalma, 4/e, pp 61–62. Hardman and Limbird, 9/e, p 21.*) The fraction of a drug dose absorbed after oral administration is affected by a wide variety of factors that can strongly influence the peak blood levels and the time to peak blood concentration. The $V_d$ and the total body clearance ($V_d$ × first-order $k_e$) also are important in determining the amount of drug that reaches the target tissue. Only the area under the blood concentration-time curve, however, reflects absorption, distribution, metabolism, and excretion factors; it is the most reliable and popular method of evaluating bioavailability.

**10. The answer is d.** (*DiPalma, 4/e, pp 48, 60–62, 77. Hardman and Limbird, 9/e, pp 4–9.*) Bioavailability is defined as the fraction or percentage of a drug that becomes available to the systemic circulation following administration by any route. This takes into consideration that not all of an orally administered drug is absorbed and that a drug can be removed from the plasma and biotransformed by the liver during its initial passage through the portal circulation. A bioavailability of 25% indicates that only 20 mg of the 80-mg dose (i.e., 80 mg × 0.25 = 20 mg) reached the systemic circulation. Organ clearance can be determined by knowing the blood flow through the organ (Q) and the extraction ratio (ER) for the drug by the organ, according to the equation

$$CL_{organ} = (Q) \times (ER)$$

The extraction ratio is dependent upon the amounts of drug entering ($C_i$) and exiting ($C_o$) the organ; i.e.,

$$ER = \frac{(C_i) \times (C_o)}{(C_i)}$$

In this problem the amount of verapamil entering the liver was 76 mg (80 mg × 0.95) and the amount leaving was 20 mg. Therefore,

$$ER = \frac{76 \text{ mg} - 20 \text{ mg}}{76 \text{ mg}} = 0.74$$

$$CL_{liver} = (1500 \text{ mL/min})(0.74) = 1110 \text{ mL/min}$$

**11. The answer is a.** (*AMA Drug Evaluations Annual 1994, pp 4, 10–11, 14–15.*) When a new chemical entity is first synthesized by a pharmaceutical company, it is given a *chemical name*, e.g., acetylsalicylic acid. During the process of investigation of the usefulness of the new chemical as a drug, it is given a *generic name* by the United States Adopted Names (USAN) Council, which negotiates with the pharmaceutical manufacturer in the choice of a meaningful and distinctive generic name for the new drug. This name will be the established, official name that can only be applied to that one unique drug compound, e.g., aspirin. The *trade name* (or *brand name*, or *proprietary name*) is a registered name given to the product by the pharmaceutical company that is manufacturing or distributing the drug and identifies a particular product containing that drug, e.g., Ecotrin. Thus, *acetylsalicylic acid, aspirin,* and *Ecotrin,* for example, all refer to the same therapeutic drug entity; however, only *aspirin* is the official generic name.

**12. The answer is c.** *(DiPalma, 4/e, pp 29–40. Hardman and Limbird, 9/e, pp 31–34.)* There are four major classes of receptors: (1) ion channel receptors, (2) receptors coupled to G proteins, (3) receptors with tyrosine-specific kinase activity, and (4) receptors for steroid hormones. In most cases, drugs that act via receptors do so by binding to extracellular receptors that transduce the information intracellularly by a variety of mechanisms. Activated ion channel receptors enhance the influx of extracellular ions into the cell; for example, the nicotinic-II cholinergic receptor selectively opens a channel for sodium ions and the GABA$_A$ receptor functions as an ionophore for chloride ions. Receptors coupled to guanine nucleotide-binding proteins (G proteins) act either by opening an ion channel or by stimulating or inhibiting specific enzymes (e.g., β-adrenergic receptor stimulation leads to an increase in cellular adenylate cyclase activity). When stimulated, receptors with tyrosine-specific protein kinase activity activate this enzyme to enhance the transport of ions and nutrients across the cell membrane; for example, insulin receptors function in this manner and increase glucose transport into insulin-dependent tissues. Steroid hormone receptors are different from all the above in that they are associated with the nucleus of the cell and are activated by steroid hormones (e.g., hydrocortisone) that penetrate into target cells. These receptors interact with DNA to enhance genetic transcription.

**13. The answer is c.** *(DiPalma, 4/e, pp 77–78. Katzung, 7/e, pp 41–42.)* Drug absorption can vary significantly depending upon the product formulation used and the route of administration. The degree to which a drug achieves a particular concentration in the blood following administration by a route other than IV injection is a measure of its efficiency of absorption—its bioavailability. When a drug is produced by different processes (e.g., at different manufacturing sites or using different manufacturing or production techniques) or in a different dosage form (e.g., capsule, tablet, suspension) and contains the same amount of active ingredient and is to be used for the same therapeutic purpose, the extent to which the bioavailability of one dosage form differs from that of another must be evaluated. In the body, these dosage forms should produce similar blood or plasma concentration-time curves. The comparison of the bioavailability of two such dosage forms is called *bioequivalence.*

The bioequivalence of different preparations is assessed by an evaluation of three parameters: (1) the peak height concentration achieved by the drug in the dosage form, (2) the time to reach the peak concentration of the drug, and (3) the area under the concentration-time curve. The ascending limb of the curve is considered to be a general reflection of the rate of drug absorption from the dosage form. The descending limb of the concentration-time curve is a general indication of the rate of elimination of the drug from the body.

None of the other choices in the question (i.e., potency, effectiveness, or plasma protein binding) can be evaluated using this type of comparison.

**14. The answer is d.** (*DiPalma, 4/e, pp 45–46. Hardman and Limbird, 9/e, pp 3–4.*) Drugs can be transferred across biologic membranes by passive processes (i.e., filtration and simple diffusion) and by specialized processes (i.e., active transport, facilitated diffusion, and pinocytosis). Active transport is a carrier-mediated process that shows all the characteristics listed in the question. Facilitated diffusion is similar to active transport except that the drug is *not* transported against a concentration gradient and *no* energy is required for this carrier-mediated system to function. Pinocytosis usually involves transport of proteins and macromolecules by a complex process in which a cell engulfs the compound within a membrane-bound vesicle.

**15. The answer is e.** (*DiPalma, 4/e, pp 52–54. Hardman and Limbird, 9/e, pp 16–17.*) The amounts of drugs excreted in milk are small compared with those excreted by other routes; but drugs in milk may have significant, undesired pharmacologic effects on breast-fed infants. The principal route of excretion of the products of a given drug varies with the drug. Some drugs are predominantly excreted by the kidneys, whereas others leave the body in the bile and feces. Inhalation anesthetic agents are eliminated by the lungs. The path of excretion may affect the clinical choice of a drug, as is the case with renal failure or hepatic insufficiency.

**16. The answer is d.** (*DiPalma, 4/e, pp 65–72. Hardman and Limbird, 9/e, pp 11–16.*) Biotransformation reactions involving the oxidation, reduction, or hydrolysis of a drug are classified as phase I (or nonsynthetic) reactions; these chemical reactions may result in either the activation or inactivation of a pharmacologic agent. There are many types of these reactions; oxidations are the most numerous. Phase II (or synthetic) reactions, which almost always result in the formation of an inactive product, involve conjugation of the drug (or its derivative) with an amino acid, carbohydrate, acetate, or sulfate. The conjugated form(s) of the drug or its derivatives may be more easily excreted than the parent compound.

**17. The answer is e.** (*DiPalma, 4/e, p 47.*) Tasteless enteric-coated tablets and capsules are formulated to resist the acidic pH found in the stomach. Once the preparation has passed into the intestine, the coating dissolves in the alkaline milieu and releases the drug. Therefore, gastric irritation, drug destruction by gastric acid, and the forming of complexes of the drug with food constituents will be avoided.

**18. The answer is e.** (*DiPalma, 4/e, pp 20–21, 28–30. Hardman and Limbird, 9/e, pp 31–34.*) Based upon the molecular mechanisms with which receptors transduce signals, four major classes of receptors have been identified: (1) ion channel receptors, (2) receptors that interact with G proteins, (3) receptors with tyrosine kinase activity, and (4) nuclear receptors. The first three types of receptors are complex membrane-bound proteins with hydrophilic regions located within the lipoid cell membrane and hydrophilic portions found protruding into the cytoplasm of the cell and the extracellular milieu; when activated, all of these receptors transmit (or transduce) information presented at the extracellular surface into ionic or biochemical signals within the cell, i.e., second messengers. Nuclear receptors are found in the nucleus of the cell, not bound to plasma membranes. In addition, these receptors do not transduce information by second messenger systems; rather, they bind to nuclear chromatin and elicit a biologic response through the transcription of DNA and alterations in the formation of cellular proteins.

Ligand binding to all types of receptors may involve the formation of ionic, hydrogen, hydrophobic, Van der Waals, and covalent bonds. In most cases, ligand-receptor interactions are stereospecific; for example, natural (−)-epinephrine is 1000 times more potent than (+)-epinephrine.

**19. The answer is e.** (*DiPalma, 4/e, pp 51–52. Hardman and Limbird, 9/e, pp 10–11.*) Since only the free (unbound) fraction of drug can cross biologic membranes, binding to plasma proteins limits a drug's concentration in tissues and therefore decreases the apparent $V_d$ of the drug. Plasma protein binding will also reduce glomerular filtration of the drug since this process is highly dependent on the free drug fraction. Renal tubular secretion and biotransformation of drugs are generally not limited by plasma protein binding because these processes reduce the free drug concentration in the plasma. If a drug is avidly transported through the tubule by the secretion process or rapidly biotransformed, the rates of these processes may exceed the rate of dissociation of the drug-protein complex (in order to restore the free:bound drug ratio in plasma) and thus becomes the rate-limiting factor for drug elimination. This assumes that equilibrium conditions exist and other influences, e.g., changes in pH or the presence of other drugs, do not occur.

**20. The answer is d.** (*DiPalma, 4/e, pp 50–51. Hardman and Limbird, 9/e, pp 9–10.*) Drugs can enter the brain from the circulation by passing through the blood-brain barrier. This boundary consists of several membranes including those of the capillary wall, the glial cells closely surrounding the capillary, and the neuron. In most cases, lipid-soluble drugs diffuse through these membranes at rates related to their lipid-to-water partition coefficients. Therefore, the greater the lipid solubility of the nonionized fraction of a weak acid or base, the more freely permeable the drug is to the brain. Some drugs enter the central nervous system (CNS) through specific carrier-mediated or receptor-mediated transport processes. Carrier-mediated systems appear to be involved predominantly in the transport of a variety of nutrients through the blood-brain barrier; however, the thyroid hormone triiodothyronine and drugs such as levodopa and methyldopa, which are structural derivatives of phenylalanine, cross the blood-brain barrier via carrier-mediated transport. Receptor-mediated transport functions to permit peptide, e.g., insulin, to enter the CNS; therefore, some peptide-like drugs are believed to gain access to the brain by this mechanism. Regardless of the process by which drugs can enter the CNS, strongly ionized drugs, e.g., quaternary amines, are unable to enter the CNS from the blood.

The exit of drugs from the CNS can involve (1) diffusion across the blood-brain barrier in the reverse direction at rates determined by the lipid solubility and degree of ionization of the drug, (2) drainage from the cerebrospinal fluid (CSF) into the dural blood sinuses by flowing through the wide channels of the arachnoid villi, and (3) active transport of certain organic anions and cations from the CSF to blood across the choroid plexuses.

**21. The answer is e.** *(Gilman, 8/e, pp 4–5. Katzung, 7/e, pp 5–6.)* Weak acids and weak bases are dissociated into nonionized and ionized forms depending upon the $pK_a$ of the molecule and the pH of the environment. The nonionized form of a drug passes through cellular membranes more easily than the ionized form because it is more lipid-soluble. Thus, the rate of passive transport varies with the proportion of the drug that is nonionized. When the pH of the environment in which a weak acid or weak base drug is contained is equal to the $pK_a$, the drug is 50% dissociated. Weak acids (e.g., salicylates, barbiturates) are more readily absorbed from the stomach than from other regions of the alimentary canal because a large percentage of these weak acids are in the nonionized state. The magnitude of this effect can be estimated by applying the Henderson-Hasselbalch equation:

$$\log \left( \frac{\text{Protonated form}}{\text{Unprotonated form}} \right) = pK_a - pH$$

At an acidic pH of about 3, of the drugs in question all are weak acids except propranolol; therefore, propranolol has the greatest percentage of its molecules in the ionized form in the stomach. The higher the value of the $pK_a$, the less ionized these substances are in the stomach.

**22–24. The answers are 22-c, 23-d, 24-a.** *(DiPalma, 4/e, pp 81–82.)* A therapeutic drug interaction that reduces drug effectiveness results when two drugs with opposing pharmacologic effects are administered. For example, isoproterenol, a β-adrenergic stimulator, will antagonize the effect of propranolol, a β-adrenergic blocking agent. The combined use of amobarbital and secobarbital, both barbiturate sedative-hypnotics, represents a drug interaction that causes an *additive* (enhanced) pharmacologic response, i.e., depression of the central nervous system. The combination of the antimicrobials sulfamethoxazole and trimethoprim is an example of a very useful drug interaction in which one drug *potentiates* the effects of another.

Physical interactions result when precipitation or another change in the physical state or solubility of a drug occurs. A common physical drug interaction takes place in the mixture of oppositely charged organic molecules, e.g., cationic (benzalkonium chloride) and anionic (soap) detergents.

Chemical drug interactions result when two administered substances combine with each other chemically. Tetracyclines complex with Ca (in milk), with aluminum (Al) and magnesium (Mg) (often components of antacids), and with Fe (in some multiple vitamins) to reduce the absorption of the tetracycline antibiotic.

**25–27. The answers are 25-e, 26-b, 27-a.** (*DiPalma, 4/e, pp 126, 375.* *Katzung, 7/e, p 132.*) Anaphylaxis refers to an acute hypersensitivity reaction that appears to be mediated primarily by immunoglobulin E (IgE). Specific antigens can interact with these antibodies and cause sensitized mast cells to release vasoactive substances, such as histamine. Anaphylaxis to penicillin is one of the best known examples; the drug of choice to relieve the symptoms is epinephrine.

Decreased sensitivity to a drug, or tolerance, is seen with some drugs such as opiates and usually requires repeated administration of the drug. Tachyphylaxis, in contrast, is tolerance that develops rapidly, often after a single injection of a drug. In some cases this may be due to what is termed the *down regulation* of a drug receptors, in which the number of receptors becomes decreased.

A person who responds to an unusually low dose of a drug is called *hyperreactive*. Supersensitivity refers to increased responses to low doses only after denervation of an organ. At least three mechanisms are responsible for supersensitivity: increased receptors, reduction in tonic neuronal activity, and decreased neurotransmitter uptake mechanisms.

**28–30. The answers are 28-c, 29-a, 30-h.** (*DiPalma, 4/e, pp 19–20.*) Time-action curves relate the changes in intensity of the action of a drug dose and the times that these changes occur. There are three distinct phases that characterize the time-action pattern of most drugs: (1) The *time to onset of action* is from the moment of administration (T on the figure that accompanies the question) to the time when the first drug effect is detected (U). (2) The *time to reach the peak effect* is from administration (T) until the maximum effect has occurred (W), regardless of whether this is above or below the level that produces some toxic effect. (3) The *duration of action* is described as the time from the appearance of a drug effect (U) until the effect disappears (Y). For some drugs a fourth phase occurs (interval Y to Z), in which *residual effects* of the drug may be present. These are usually undetectable, but may be uncovered by readministration of the same drug dose (observed as an increase in potency) or by administration of another drug (leading to some drug-drug interaction).

**31–33. The answers are 31-b, 32-a, 33-d.** (*DiPalma, 4/e, pp 45–46.*) The absorption, distribution, and elimination of drugs require that they cross various cellular membranes. The descriptions given in the question define the various transport mechanisms. The most common method by which ionic compounds of low molecular weight (100 to 200) enter cells is via membrane channels. The degree to which such filtration occurs varies from cell type to cell type because their pore sizes differ.

Simple diffusion is another mechanism by which substances cross membranes without the active participation of components in the membranes. Generally, lipid-soluble substances employ this method to enter cells. Both simple diffusion and filtration are dominant factors in most drug absorption, distribution, and elimination.

Pinocytosis is a type of endocytosis that is responsible for the transport of large molecules such as proteins and colloids. Some cell types—for example, endothelial cells—employ this transport mechanism extensively, but its importance in drug action is uncertain.

Membrane carriers are proteinaceous components of the cell membrane that are capable of combining with a drug at one surface of the membrane. The carrier-solute complex moves across the membrane, the solute is released, and the carrier then returns to the original surface where it can combine with another molecule of solute. There are two primary types of carrier-mediated transport: *active transport* and *facilitated diffusion*. During active transport (1) the drug crosses the membrane against a concentration gradient, (2) the transport mechanism becomes saturated at high drug concentrations and thus shows a *transport maximum*, and (3) the process is selective for certain structural configurations of the drug. Active transport is responsible for the movement of a number of organic acids and bases across membranes of renal tubules, choroid plexuses, and hepatic cells. With facilitated diffusion, the transport process is selective and saturable, but the drug is *not* transferred against a concentration gradient and does *not* require the expenditure of cellular energy. Glucose transport into erythrocytes is a good example of this process. In both situations, if two compounds are transported by the same mechanism, one will competitively inhibit the transport of the other and the transport process can be inhibited noncompetitively by substances that interfere with cellular metabolism.

**34–36. The answers are 34-g, 35-a, 36-d.** (*DiPalma, 4/e, pp 66–69. Katzung, 7/e, pp 52–55.*) There are four major components to the mixed-function oxidase system: (1) cytochrome P-450, (2) NADPH, or reduced nicotinamide adenine dinucleotide phosphate, (3) NADPH–cytochrome P-450 reductase, and (4) molecular oxygen. The figure that follows shows the catalytic cycle for the reactions dependent upon cytochrome P-450.

Cytochrome P-450 catalyzes a diverse number of oxidative reactions involved in drug biotransformation; it undergoes reduction and oxidation during its catalytic cycle. A prosthetic group composed of Fe and protoporphyrin IX (forming heme) binds molecular oxygen and converts it to an "activated" form for interaction with the drug substrate. Similar to hemoglobin, cytochrome P-450 is inhibited by carbon monoxide. This interaction results in an absorbance spectrum peak at 450 nm, hence the name *P-450*.

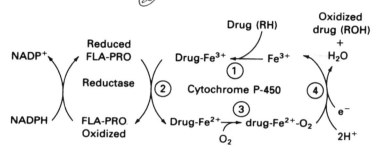

(From DiPalma and DiGregorio, with permission.)

NADPH gives up hydrogen atoms to the flavoprotein NADPH–cytochrome P-450 reductase and becomes NADP+. The reduced flavoprotein transfers these reducing equivalents to cytochrome P-450. The reducing equivalents are used to activate molecular oxygen for incorporation into the substrate, as described above. Thus NADPH provides the reducing equivalents, while NADPH–cytochrome P-450 reductase passes them on to the catalytic enzyme cytochrome P-450.

MAO is a flavoprotein enzyme that is found on the outer membrane of mitochondria. It oxidatively deaminates short-chain monoamines only and it is not part of the DMMS. ATP is involved in transfer of reducing equivalents through the mitochondrial respiratory chain, not the microsomal system.

# ANTI-INFECTIVES

**Note: In the classification of drugs, prototype drugs are marked with an asterisk (*).**

General Concepts: β-Lactam
  Antibiotics
  1) Cell-wall synthesis
  2) Inhibition by β-lactam
    antibiotics
  Autolytic enzyme activity
    Autolysin-deficient bacteria
  Penicillin-binding proteins
    (PBPs)
  Mechanisms of resistance
    Permeability barrier
    β-Lactamase production
Penicillins
  Natural penicillins
    Penicillin G*
    Penicillin V
  Penicillinase-resistant
    Methacillin
    Nafcillin
    Oxacillin
    Cloxacillin
    Dicloxacillin
  Aminopenicillins
    Ampicillin*
    Amoxicillin
  Extended-spectrum
    Carbenicillin
    Ticarcillin
    Azlocillin

Mezlocillin
Piperacillin
β-Lactamase Inhibitors
  Clavulanic acid*
  Sulbactam
  Tazobactam
Cephalosporins
  First generation
    Parenteral use
    Cefazolin
    Cephalothin*
    Cephapirin
    Cephradine
    Oral use
    Cephalexin*
    Cefadroxil
    Cephradine
  Second generation
    Parenteral use
    Cefuroxime*
    Cefonicid
    Cefmetazole
    Cefoxitin
    Cefotetan
    Oral use
    Cefaclor*
    Cefuroxime*
    Cefprozil
    Loracarbef

Third generation
  Parenteral use
    Ceftazidime
    Cefotaxime*
    Ceftizoxime
    Cefoperazone
    Ceftriaxone
  Oral use
    Cefixime
    Cefpodoxime proxetil
  Carbapenems
    Imipenem-cilastatin
  Monobactams
    Aztreonam
Miscellaneous Antibiotics
  Primarily against Gram-positives
    Azithromycin
    Erythromycin*
    Clarithromycin*
    Vancomycin*
  Primarily against anaerobes
    Clindamycin*
    Metronidazole*
  Primarily against Gram-negatives
    Streptomycin*
    Gentamicin
    Tobramycin
    Amikacin
    Netilmicin
    Ciprofloxacin
    Norfloxacin
    Enoxacin
    Ofloxacin
    Lomefloxacin
  Primarily for *Neisseria gonorrhoeae*
    Spectinomycin (not an amino-
      glycoside)

Broad-Spectrum Antimicrobials
  Chloramphenicol*
  Clindamycin
  Metronidazole
  Tetracyclines*
    Tetracycline
    Oxytetracycline
    Demeclocycline
    Methacycline
    Doxycycline
    Minocycline
  Sulfonamides
    Sulfisoxazole
    Sulfadiazine*
    Sulfamethoxazole
    Sulfamerazine
    Sulfamethazine
    Sulfamethizole
    Sulfameter
    Sulfadoxine
  Trimethoprim*
  Trimethoprim-
    sulfamethoxazole*
Antituberculosis drugs
  Isoniazid*
  Rifampin*
  Ethambutol*
  Pyrazinamide
  Streptomycin*
  Ethionamide
  Capreomycin
  Kanamycin
  Para-aminosalicylic
    acid (PAS)
Drugs for leprosy
  Dapsone*
  Clofazimine

Antimycotic drugs
Amphotericin B*
Nystatin*
Flucytosine*
Griseofulvin*
Ketoconazole*
Miconazole
Butoconazole
Oxiconazole
Antiviral drugs
Amantadine*
Acyclovir*
Vidarabine
Trifluridine
Idoxuridine*
Ribavirin
Zidovudine*
Protozoan infections
Malaria
Quinine, mefloquine*
Chloroquine*
Primaquine*
Proguanil
Pyrimethamine*
Trimethoprim
Sulfonamides
Qinghaosu, artemisinine
Amebiasis
Diloxanide furoate*
Metronidazole*
Tinidazole
Emetine*
Dehydroemetine
Iodoquinol*
Paromomycin

Carbarsone
Chloroquine
Leishmaniasis
Sodium stibogluconate*
Amphotericin B*
Metronidazole*
Allopurinol
Nifurtimox
Trypanosomiasis
Pentamidine
Melarsoprol
Nifurtimox
Suramin
Giardiasis
Metronidazole*
Quinacrine
Furazolidone
Trichomoniasis
Metronidazole*
Toxoplasmosis
Pyrimethamine-sulfadiazine
Pneumonia caused by
*Pneumocystis carinii*
Trimethoprim-sulfamethoxazole
Pentamidine
Antihelminthics
Mebendazole
Diethylcarbamazine
Pyrantel
Thiabendazole
Piperazine
Quinacrine
Niclosamide
Oxamniquine
Praziquantel

# Questions

**DIRECTIONS:** Each question below contains several suggested responses. Select the **one best** response to each question.

**37.** A 19-year-old male being treated for leukemia develops fever. You give agents that will cover bacterial, viral, and fungal infections. Two days later, he develops acute renal failure. Which drug was most likely responsible?

a. vancomycin
b. ceftazidime
c. amphotericin B
d. acyclovir

**38.** A 26-year-old female with acquired immunodeficiency syndrome (AIDS) develops cryptococcal meningitis. She refuses all intravenous (IV) medication. Which antifungal agent can be given orally to treat the meningeal infection?

a. ketoconazole
b. amphotericin B
c. fluconazole
d. nystatin

**39.** Why is vitamin B6 usually prescribed with isoniazid (INH)?

a. it acts as a cofactor for INH
b. it prevents some adverse effects of INH therapy
c. like INH, it has tuberculostatic activity
d. it prevents metabolism of INH

**40.** The quinolone derivative effective against *Pseudomonas aeruginosa* is

a. norfloxacin
b. ciprofloxacin
c. ofloxacin
d. enoxacin
e. lomefloxacin

**41.** A 19-year-old woman is diagnosed with tuberculosis (TB). Before prescribing a drug regimen, you take a careful medication history because one of the drugs commonly used to treat TB induces microsomal cytochrome P-450 enzymes in the liver. Which drug is this?

a. isoniazid
b. rifampin
c. pyrazinamide
d. ethambutol
e. vitamin B6

**42.** The elimination half-life of which of the following tetracyclines remains unchanged when the drug is administered to an anuric patient?

a. methacycline
b. oxytetracycline
c. doxycycline
d. tetracycline
e. none of the above

**43.** In the treatment of bacterial meningitis in children, the drug of choice is

a. penicillin G
b. penicillin V
c. erythromycin
d. procaine penicillin
e. ceftriaxone

**44.** In patients with hepatic coma, decreases in the production and absorption of ammonia from the gastrointestinal (GI) tract will be beneficial. The antibiotic of choice in this situation would be

a. neomycin
b. tetracycline
c. penicillin G
d. chloramphenicol
e. cephalothin

**45.** Indicate from the diagram below the site of action of penicillinase.

a. A
b. B
c. C
d. D
e. E

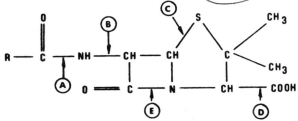

**46.** Clavulanic acid is important because it

a. easily penetrates Gram-negative microorganisms
b. is specific for Gram-positive microorganisms
c. is a potent inhibitor of cell wall transpeptidase
d. inactivates bacterial β-lactamases
e. has a spectrum of activity similar to that of penicillin G

**47.** In the treatment of infections caused by *P. aeruginosa*, the antimicrobial agent that has proved to be effective is

a. penicillin G
b. piperacillin
c. nafcillin
d. erythromycin
e. tetracycline

**48.** Ethambutol is administered concurrently with other antitubercular drugs in the treatment of TB in order to

a.  reduce the pain of injection
b.  facilitate penetration of the blood-brain barrier
c.  retard the development of organism resistance
d.  delay excretion of other antitubercular drugs by the kidney
e.  retard absorption after intramuscular (IM) injection

**49.** The most active aminoglycoside against *Mycobacterium tuberculosis* is

a.  streptomycin
b.  amikacin
c.  neomycin
d.  tobramycin
e.  kanamycin

**50.** The drug used in all types of TB is

a.  ethambutol
b.  cycloserine
c.  streptomycin
d.  INH
e.  PAS

**51.** Chronic candidiasis infections of the GI tract and oral cavity are treated orally with

a.  amphotericin B
b.  nystatin
c.  miconazole
d.  fluconazole
e.  clotrimazole

**52.** Drug X is an antimycobacterial agent that inhibits other bacteria as well as poxviruses. However, it should not be used as a single agent because resistant mutants frequently form. The responsible mutation may alter the site of action of drug X; that is, the deoxyribonucleic acid (DNA)-dependent ribonucleic acid (RNA) polymerase. What is drug X?

a.  INH
b.  rifampin
c.  pyrazinamide
d.  ethambutol

**53.** For the treatment of a patient with *Legionella pneumophilia,* the drug of choice would be

a.  penicillin G
b.  chloramphenicol
c.  erythromycin
d.  streptomycin
e.  lincomycin

**54.** The most effective agent in the treatment of *Rickettsia, Mycoplasma,* and *Chlamydia* infections is

a.  penicillin G
b.  tetracycline
c.  vancomycin
d.  gentamicin
e.  bacitracin

**55.** The mechanism of action by which pyrantel pamoate is effective for the treatment of *Necator americanus* (hookworm) disease is

a.  interference with cell-wall synthesis
b.  interference with cell division
c.  inhibition of neuromuscular transmission
d.  interference with protein synthesis
e.  depletion of membrane lipoproteins

**56.** Vertigo, inability to perceive termination of movement, and difficulty in sitting or standing without visual clues are some of the toxic reactions that are likely to occur in about 75% of patients who

a. are allergic to penicillin
b. receive tetracycline therapy
c. receive amphotericin B therapy
d. receive streptomycin therapy
e. receive INH therapy for TB

**57.** Amantadine, a synthetic antiviral agent used prophylactically against influenza $A_2$, is thought to act by

a. preventing production of viral capsid protein
b. preventing virion release
c. preventing penetration of the virus into the host cell
d. preventing synthesis of nucleic acid
e. causing lysis of infected host cells by release of intracellular lysosomal enzymes

**58.** Streptomycin and other aminoglycosides inhibit bacterial protein synthesis by binding

a. peptidoglycan units in the cell wall
b. messenger RNA (mRNA)
c. DNA
d. 30S ribosomal particles
e. RNA polymerase

**59.** Which of the following statements concerning griseofulvin is true?

a. it inhibits the growth of dermatophytes
b. it inhibits synthesis of the cell wall
c. it inhibits synthesis of the cell membrane
d. it is used primarily as a short-term drug
e. it is administered primarily by the parenteral route

**60.** A 39-year-old male with gastroenteritis and no drug allergies is given an IV dose of antibiotic at a fast rate. As the antibiotic is infusing, the patient becomes flushed over most of his body. What antibiotic was given?

a. vancomycin
b. gentamicin
c. erythromycin
d. penicillin G
e. tetracycline

**61.** Which of the following cephalosporins would have increased activity against anaerobic bacteria such as *Bacteroides fragilis?*

a. cefaclor
b. cephalothin
c. cephalexin
d. cefamandole
e. cefoxitin

**62.** Which one of the following antimicrobial agents is primarily administered topically?

a. polymyxin B
b. penicillin G
c. dicloxacillin
d. carbenicillin
e. streptomycin

**63.** A 75-year-old woman is hospitalized for pneumonia and treated with an IV antibiotic. On day three, she develops severe diarrhea. Stool is positive for *Clostridium difficile* toxin. What is the best treatment?

a.   clindamycin
b.   cefaclor
c.   vancomycin
d.   erythromycin

**64.** A jaundiced one-day-old premature infant with an elevated free bilirubin is seen in the premature-baby nursery. The mother received an antibiotic combination preparation containing sulfamethizole for a urinary tract infection (UTI) one week before delivery. You suspect that the infant's findings are caused by the sulfonamide because of the following mechanism:

a.   enhanced synthesis of bilirubin
b.   competition between the sulfonamide and bilirubin for binding sites on albumin
c.   inhibition of bilirubin degradation
d.   inhibition of urinary excretion of bilirubin

**65.** A 27-year-old female has just returned from a trip to Southeast Asia. In the past 24 hours, she has developed shaking, chills, and a temperature of 104°F. A blood smear reveals *Plasmodium vivax*. Which of the following agents is the drug of choice?

a.   primaquine
b.   pyrimethamine
c.   quinacrine
d.   chloroquine
e.   chloroguanide

**66.** An 86-year-old male complains of cough and blood in his sputum for the past two days. On admission, his temperature is 103°F. Physical examination reveals rales in his right lung, and x-ray examination shows increased density in the right middle lobe. A sputum smear shows many Gram-positive cocci, confirmed by sputum culture as penicillinase-producing *Staphylococcus aureus*. Which of the following agents should be given?

a.   ampicillin
b.   oxacillin
c.   carbenicillin
d.   ticarcillin
e.   mezlocillin

**67.** A 40-year-old male is HIV-positive with a cluster of differentiation 4 (CD4) count of 200/mm$^3$. Within two months, he develops a peripheral white blood cell count of 1000/mm$^3$ and a hemoglobin of 9.0 mg/dL. Which drug has most likely caused the adverse effect?

a.  acyclovir
b.  dideoxycytidine
c.  foscarnet
d.  rimantadine
e.  zidovudine

**68.** Thiabendazole, a benzimidazole derivative, is an antihelminthic drug used primarily to treat infections caused by

a.  *Ascaris lumbricoides* (roundworm)
b.  *N. americanus* (hookworm)
c.  *Strongyloides*
d.  *Enterobius vermicularis*
e.  *Taenia saginata* (flatworm)

**69.** A 30-year-old male with a two-year history of chronic renal failure requiring dialysis consents to transplantation. A donor kidney becomes available. He is given cyclosporine to prevent transplant rejection just before surgery. What is the most likely adverse effect of this drug?

a.  bone marrow depression
b.  nephrotoxicity
c.  oral and GI ulceration
d.  pancreatitis
e.  seizures

**70.** The mechanism of action of chloroquine in *Plasmodium falciparum* malaria is elimination of

a.  secondary tissue schizonts
b.  exoerythrocytic schizonts
c.  the erythrocytic stage
d.  asexual forms
e.  sporozoites

**71.** The use of chloramphenicol may result in

a.  bone marrow stimulation
b.  phototoxicity
c.  aplastic anemia
d.  staining of teeth
e.  alopecia

**72.** A drug primarily used in pneumonia caused by *Pneumocystis carinii* is

a.  nifurtimox
b.  penicillin G
c.  metronidazole
d.  pentamidine
e.  carbenicillin

Antiparasitic → Drug of choice

**DIRECTIONS:** Each group of questions below consists of lettered headings followed by a set of numbered items. For each numbered item select the one lettered heading with which it is **most** closely associated.

**Questions 73–75**

For each patient, select the mechanism of drug action:

a. inhibition of bacterial cell wall synthesis
b. inhibition of bacterial protein synthesis
c. inhibition of bacterial folic acid synthesis
d. inhibition of bacterial topoisomerase II (DNA gyrase)
e. inhibition of bacterial DNA polymerase

**73.** A 39-year-old female with a history of chronic UTI develops a new infection with *Escherichia coli* that is sensitive to norfloxacin.

**74.** A 25-year-old female with a sinus infection caused by *Haemophilus influenzae* is treated with trimethoprim-sulfamethoxazole.

**75.** A 35-year-old male has recently converted to positive on a purified protein derivative of tuberculin (PPD) test for TB. INH is given as prophylaxis.

**76.** Neuromuscular blockade produced by tubocurarine is potentiated by

a. neomycin
b. bacitracin
c. cephalothin
d. penicillin
e. chloramphenicol

**77.** Chloramphenicol, a completely synthetic antibiotic, is the drug of choice in

a. symptomatic *Salmonella* infections
b. brucellosis
c. UTI by *E. coli*
d. cholera
e. streptococcal pharyngitis

**78.** Which of the following best describes cimetidine's mechanism of interaction with ketoconazole?

a. it decreases ketoconazole metabolism
b. it decreases ketoconazole sensitivity at the site of action
c. it decreases ketoconazole renal excretion
d. it decreases ketoconazole plasma protein binding
e. it decreases ketoconazole intestinal absorption

**79.** Of the following, the most appropriate statement concerning the reactions caused by aminoglycosides is that these agents

a. produce ototoxicity
b. are potent neuromuscular blockers
c. have little or no effect on kidneys
d. produce a high incidence of hypersensitivity reactions similar to those of penicillins
e. produce a high incidence of exfoliative dermatitis

## Questions 80–81

For each patient, select the drug that most likely caused the adverse effect:

a. acyclovir
b. amantadine
c. dideoxycytidine
d. foscarnet
e. ganciclovir
f. idoxuridine
g. interferon α
h. ribavirin
i. vidarabine
j. zidovudine

**80.** A 27-year-old male with a three-year history of AIDS complains of progressive blurring of vision for two days. Eye examination reveals evidence of retinitis consistent with cytomegalic virus inclusion disease. IV treatment is started, and within five days the patient complains of muscular weakness and cramping. Blood chemistries show a creatinine of 5.2 mEq/L and a Ca of 6.9 mEq/L.

**81.** A 22-year-old female with a two-year history of AIDS treated with one of these agents develops epigastric pain that radiates to the chest. Endoscopic examination reveals an esophageal ulceration.

**82.** The mechanism of action of chloramphenicol as an antibiotic is that it

a. binds to the 30S ribosome subunit
b. reversibly binds to the 50S ribosome subunit
c. prevents cell-membrane development
d. inhibits cell-wall synthesis
e. inhibits RNA polymerase

**83.** The drug of choice for the treatment of *T. saginata* (tapeworm) is

a. praziquantel
b. ceftriaxone
c. primaquine
d. niclosamide
e. chloroquine

**84.** The drug of choice for the treatment of *Schistosoma haematobium* is

a. praziquantel
b. ceftriaxone
c. metronidazole
d. mebendazole
e. diethylcarbamazine

**85.** Ampicillin and amoxicillin are in the same group of penicillins. Which of the following statements best characterizes amoxicillin?

a. it has better oral absorption than does ampicillin
b. it can be used in penicillinase-producing organisms
c. it is classified as a broad-spectrum penicillin
d. it does not cause hypersensitivity reactions
e. it is effective against *Pseudomonas*

**DIRECTIONS:** Each numbered question or incomplete statement below is NEGATIVELY phrased. Select the **one best** lettered response.

**86.** All the following agents are β-lactam antibiotics EXCEPT

a. penicillins
b. cephalosporins
c. monobactams
d. quinolones
e. carbapenems

**87.** All the following are properties of amphotericin B EXCEPT

a. it can cause renal and liver dysfunctions
b. it is poorly absorbed via the oral route
c. it is used for the treatment of systemic fungal infections
d. it binds to ergosterol to disturb the fungal membrane
e. it is a potent inhibitor of cell-wall synthesis

**88.** All the following antibiotics inhibit bacterial cell-wall synthesis EXCEPT

a. bacitracin
b. cycloserine
c. cephalothin
d. vancomycin
e. polymyxins

**89.** All the following penicillins are resistant to penicillinase EXCEPT

a. oxacillin
b. cloxacillin
c. ticarcillin
d. nafcillin
e. dicloxacillin

**90.** Quinine, an antimalarial drug, causes all the following EXCEPT

a. local anesthesia
b. local destruction of tissue
c. analgesia
d. antipyretic effects
e. hypertension

**91.** Idoxuridine is a synthetic antiviral agent with all the following properties EXCEPT

a. a structure containing a halogen atom
b. activity against DNA viruses
c. major use in the treatment of herpes simplex keratitis
d. topical use on the eye
e. major use in treatment of herpes simplex virus type 2

**92.** All the following are associated with the use of penicillin EXCEPT

a. hypersensitization
b. interstitial nephritis
c. impaired platelet function
d. seizures
e. disulfiram-like reaction

**93.** All the following statements are true concerning cephalosporins in comparison with penicillins EXCEPT

a.  their structures are closely related
b.  their mechanisms of action are analogous
c.  cephalosporins have an unusually broader antimicrobial spectrum
d.  their hypersensitivity reactions are distinguished by distinct signs and symptoms
e.  cephalosporins can cause bleeding problems related to hypoprothrombinemia

**94.** All the following statements are associated with the antibiotic methicillin EXCEPT (MRSA)

a.  it causes hypersensitivity
b.  it is administered only orally
c.  it is resistant to penicillinase
d.  it causes interstitial nephritis
e.  it is poorly bound to serum proteins

**95.** Metronidazole is effective in the treatment of all the following EXCEPT

a.  trichomoniasis in females
b.  asymptomatic trichomoniasis in males
c.  giardiasis
d.  infection with B. fragilis
e.  streptococcal infection

**96.** Common complications of cephalothin therapy in hospitalized patients include all the following EXCEPT

a.  fever, eosinophilia, and anaphylaxis
b.  superinfection with Gram-negative organisms
c.  thrombophlebitis
d.  nephrotoxicity
e.  hemolytic anemia

**97.** All the following statements are true of acyclovir EXCEPT

a.  it is a nucleoside antiviral drug
b.  it converts to a triphosphate and subsequently inhibits synthesis of viral DNA
c.  it is available topically and orally
d.  it is used against herpes simplex
e.  it is an analogue of purine metabolites

**98.** By certain changes in the side chain of penicillin structure, the pharmacology is markedly altered. Carbenicillin has all the following properties EXCEPT

a.  it is classified as an aminopenicillin
b.  it is given only parenterally
c.  it is sensitive to penicillinase
d.  it is effective against most Gram-negative organisms
e.  in combination with an aminoglycoside, it exhibits increased activity against Pseudomonas

**99.** A 44-year-old male with a five-year history of using calcium ($Ca^{++}$)- and magnesium ($Mg^{++}$)-containing antacids for peptic ulcer disease develops acute bronchitis with sputum production. Of the broad-spectrum antibiotics listed, which would NOT be easily absorbed?

a.  ampicillin
b.  chloramphenicol
c.  norfloxacin
d.  tetracycline
e.  sulfamethoxazole-trimethoprim

**DIRECTIONS:** Each group of questions below consists of lettered headings followed by a set of numbered items. For each numbered item select the one lettered heading with which it is **most** closely associated. Each lettered heading may be used **once, more than once, or not at all.**

## Questions 100–102

For each of the parasites below, select the drug that is most effective against it.

a. bithionol
b. methotrexate
c. pyrantel pamoate
d. penicillin
e. praziquantel
f. ceftriaxone
g. diethylcarbamazine
h. primaquine
i. niclosamide
j. chloroquine

**100.** *A. lumbricoides* (roundworms)

**101.** *Wuchereria bancrofti* (filariae)

**102.** *Fasciola hepatica* (sheep liver flukes)

## Questions 103–105

For each of the drugs below, select the most suitable description.

a. parenteral penicillin that is resistant to β-lactamase
b. oral penicillin that is resistant to β-lactamase
c. referred to as an extended-spectrum penicillin
d. chemically a cephalosporin
e. related to ampicillin but with better oral absorption
f. administered IM and yields prolonged drug levels
g. cause of a disulfiram-like reaction
h. given parenterally and may cause elevation of serum sodium
i. cause of hypothrombinemia

**103.** Benzathine penicillin G

**104.** Methicillin

**105.** Piperacillin

# ANTI-INFECTIVES

## Answers

**37. The answer is c.** (*Hardman and Limbird, 9/e, p 1179. Katzung, 7/e, p 781.*) Amphotericin B may alter kidney function by decreasing creatinine clearance; if this occurs, the dose must be reduced. It also commonly increases potassium (K) clearance, leading to hypokalemia, and causes anemia and neurologic symptoms. A liposomal preparation may reduce the incidence of renal and neurologic toxicity. Vancomycin is less likely to cause kidney damage; if it does, the damage is less severe.

**38. The answer is c.** (*Hardman and Limbird, 9/e, p 1183. Katzung, 7/e, p 785.*) Fluconazole penetrates into cerebrospinal fluid, where it is active against *Cryptococcus neoformans*. When it is given orally, blood levels are almost as high as when it is given parenterally.

**39. The answer is b.** (*Hardman and Limbird, 9/e, p 1158.*) INH inhibits cell wall synthesis in mycobacteria. Increasing vitamin B6 levels prevents complications associated with this inhibition, including peripheral neuritis, insomnia, restlessness, muscle twitching, urinary retention, convulsions, and psychosis, without affecting the antimycobacterial activity of INH.

**40. The answer is b.** (*DiPalma, 4/e, pp 724–725. Hardman and Limbird, 9/e, p 1065.*) Ciprofloxacin is a fluorinated quinolone derivative highly effective against *P. aeruginosa*. Other derivatives in this class have little or no activity toward this organism, although they are effective against other common Gram-negative organisms.

**41. The answer is b.** (*Katzung, 7/e, p 773.*) Rifampin induces P-450 enzymes, which causes a significant increase in elimination of drugs such as oral contraceptives, anticoagulants, ketoconazole, cyclosporine, and chloramphenicol. It also promotes urinary excretion of methadone, which may precipitate withdrawal.

**42. The answer is c.** *(DiPalma, 4/e, p 745. Hardman and Limbird, 9/e, pp 1129–1131.)* All tetracyclines can produce negative nitrogen balance and increased blood urea nitrogen (BUN) levels. This is of clinical importance in patients with impaired renal function. With the exception of doxycycline, tetracyclines should not be used in patients that are anuric. Doxycycline is excreted by the GI tract under these conditions and it will not accumulate in the serum of patients with renal insufficiency.

**43. The answer is e.** *(DiPalma, 4/e, pp 712–713. Hardman and Limbird, 9/e, pp 1094–1095.)* Penicillins are rarely used in the treatment of meningitis because of their failure to pass across the blood-brain barrier. Most cephalosporins also have poor penetration into the central nervous system, but the third-generation cephalosporin ceftriaxone is highly effective against *H. influenzae* meningitis in children.

**44. The answer is a.** *(Hardman and Limbird, 9/e, pp 1116–1117.)* Neomycin, an aminoglycoside, is not significantly absorbed from the GI tract. After oral administration, the intestinal flora is suppressed or modified and the drug is excreted in the feces. This effect of neomycin is used in hepatic coma to decrease the coliform flora, thus decreasing the production of ammonia causing the levels of free nitrogen to decrease in the bloodstream. Other antimicrobial agents—such as tetracycline, penicillin G, chloramphenicol, and cephalothin—do not have the potency of neomycin in causing this effect.

**45. The answer is e.** *(DiPalma, 4/e, p 696. Hardman and Limbird, 9/e, pp 1074–1076.)* Penicillinase hydrolyzes the β-lactam ring of penicillin G to form inactive penicilloic acid. Consequently, the antibiotic is ineffective in the therapy of infections caused by penicillinase-producing microorganisms such as staphylococci, bacilli, *E. coli, P. aeruginosa,* and *M. tuberculosis.*

**46. The answer is d.** *(DiPalma, 4/e, pp 705–706. Hardman and Limbird, 9/e, pp 1097–1098.)* The antibiotic clavulanic acid is a potent inhibitor of β-lactamases. The mode of inhibition is irreversible. Although clavulanic acid does not effectively inhibit the transpeptidase, it may be used in conjunction with a β-lactamase-sensitive penicillin to potentiate its activity.

*good point*

**47. The answer is b.** (*DiPalma, 4/e, pp 704–705. Hardman and Limbird, 9/e, pp 1077–1086.*) Piperacillin is a broad-spectrum, semisynthetic penicillin for parenteral use. Its spectrum of activity includes various Gram-positive and Gram-negative organisms including *Pseudomonas.* The indications for piperacillin are similar to those for carbenicillin, ticarcillin, and mezlocillin with the primary use being suspected or proven infections caused by *P. aeruginosa.* Penicillin G, nafcillin, erythromycin, and tetracycline are ineffective against *Pseudomonas.*

**48. The answer is c.** (*DiPalma, 4/e, pp 750–751. Hardman and Limbird, 9/e, pp 1161–1162.*) An important problem in the chemotherapy of TB is bacterial drug resistance. For this reason, concurrent administration of two or more drugs should be employed to delay the development of drug resistance. Isoniazid is often combined with ethambutol for this purpose. Streptomycin or rifampin may also be added to the regimen to delay even further the development of drug resistance.

**49. The answer is a.** (*DiPalma, 4/e, pp 721–722. Hardman and Limbird, 9/e, pp 1105–1108.*) The activity of streptomycin is bactericidal for the tubercle bacillus organism. Other aminoglycosides–such as gentamicin, tobramycin, neomycin, amikacin, and kanamycin–have activity against this organism but are seldom used clinically because of toxicity or development of resistance.

**50. The answer is d.** (*DiPalma, 4/e, p 747–748. Hardman and Limbird, 9/e, pp 1155–1159.*) Isoniazid is an effective tuberculostatic drug. Only actively growing bacilli are susceptible to the bactericidal property of INH. The major action of INH is on the cell wall of the bacillus, where it prevents the synthesis of mycolic acid.

**51. The answer is d.** (*DiPalma, 4/e, pp 757, 759. Hardman and Limbird, 9/e, pp 1183–1184.*) Mucocutaneous infections, most commonly *Candida albicans,* involve the moist skin and mucous membranes. Agents used topically include amphotericin B, nystatin, miconazole, and clotrimazole. Ketoconazole and fluconazole are administered orally for treatment of chronic infections.

**52. The answer is b.** (*Hardman and Limbird, 9/e, p 1159.*) Rifampin inhibits RNA synthesis in bacteria, mycobacteria, and chlamydiae by binding to the DNA-dependent RNA polymerase; it also inhibits assembly of poxvirus particles. Rifampin is used as a single prophylactic agent for contacts of people with meningococcal or *H. influenzae* type b infections. Otherwise, it is not used alone because 1 in 10 organisms in a population exposed to rifampin will become resistant, possibly because of mutation or a barrier against rifampin's entry into cells.

**53. The answer is c.** (*DiPalma, 4/e, p 730. Hardman and Limbird, 9/e, pp 1135–1141.*) Erythromycin, a macrolide antibiotic, was initially designed to be used in penicillin-sensitive patients with streptococcal or pneumococcal infections. Erythromycin has become the drug of choice for the treatment of pneumonia caused by *Mycoplasma* and *Legionella*.

**54. The answer is b.** (*DiPalma, 4/e, pp 743–745. Hardman and Limbird, 9/e, p 1128.*) Tetracycline is one of the drugs of choice in the treatment of *Rickettsia*, *Mycoplasma*, and *Chlamydia* infections. The antibiotics that act by inhibiting cell wall synthesis have no effect on *Mycoplasma* since the organism does not possess a cell wall; penicillin G, vancomycin, and bacitracin will be ineffective. Gentamicin has little or no antimicrobial activity with these organisms.

**55. The answer is c.** (*DiPalma, 4/e, pp 794–795. Hardman and Limbird, 9/e, p 1022.*) Pyrantel pamoate is an antihelminthic that acts primarily as a depolarizing neuromuscular blocker. In certain worms, a spastic neuromuscular paralysis occurs, resulting in the expulsion of the worms from the intestinal tract of the host. Pyrantel also exerts its effect against parasites via release of acetylcholine and inhibition of cholinesterase.

**56. The answer is d.** (*DiPalma, 4/e, pp 722–723. Hardman and Limbird, 9/e, pp 1110–1113.*) Streptomycin and other aminoglycosides can elicit toxic reactions involving both the vestibular and auditory branches of the eighth cranial nerve. Patients receiving an aminoglycoside should be monitored frequently for any hearing impairment owing to the irreversible deafness that may result from its prolonged use. None of the other agents listed in the question adversely affect the function of the eighth cranial nerve.

**57. The answer is c.** (*DiPalma, 4/e, pp 764, 767. Hardman and Limbird, 9/e, pp 1209–1211.*) Amantadine's mechanism of action is not entirely understood, but it appears to block the attachment of the virus to cells. The drug does not affect penetration and RNA-dependent RNA polymerase activity. Amantadine both reduces the frequency of illness and diminishes the serologic response to influenza infection. The drug has no action, however, on influenza B. As a weak base, amantadine buffers the pH of endosomes, thus blocking the fusion of the viral envelope with the membrane of the endosome.

**58. The answer is d.** (*DiPalma, 4/e, pp 719–720. Hardman and Limbird, 9/e, pp 1105–1108.*) The bactericidal activity of streptomycin and other aminoglycosides involves a direct action on the 30S ribosomal subunit, the site at which these agents both inhibit protein synthesis and diminish the accuracy of translation of the genetic code. Proteins containing improper sequences of amino acids ("nonsense" proteins) are often nonfunctional.

**59. The answer is a.** (*DiPalma, 4/e, p 760. Hardman and Limbird, 9/e, p 1184.*) Griseofulvin is a potent, orally administered antifungal agent effective against various dermatophytes including *Epidermophyton* and *Trichophyton*. The mechanism of action appears to be related to the interference of nucleic acid synthesis and polymerization. When given for a specific fungal infection, griseofulvin must be continued for 3 to 6 weeks if only hair or skin is involved, but 3 to 6 months if nails are affected.

**60. The answer is a.** (*Hardman and Limbird, 9/e, p 1146.*) The "red man" syndrome is associated with vancomycin, thought to be caused by histamine release. Prevention consists of a slower infusion rate and pretreatment with antihistamines.

**61. The answer is e.** (*DiPalma, 4/e, p 711. Hardman and Limbird, 9/e, pp 1092–1094.*) Cefoxitin and moxalactam are suitable for treating intra-abdominal infections. Such infections are caused by mixtures of aerobic and anaerobic Gram-negative bacteria like *B. fragilis.* Cefoxitin alone has been shown to be as effective as the traditional therapy of clindamycin plus gentamicin.

**62. The answer is a.** (*Hardman and Limbird, 9/e, pp 1143–1144.*) Polymyxin B is poorly absorbed by the oral route. It is primarily administered by the topical route for the treatment of infections of the skin, mucous membranes, eye, and ear. Penicillin G can be administered both orally and parenterally. Dicloxacillin is only given by the oral route. Carbenicillin and streptomycin are administered only by the parenteral route.

**63. The answer is c.** *(Hardman and Limbird, 9/e, p 1146.)* Vancomycin is often used to treat antibiotic-associated enterocolitis, especially when caused by *C. difficile*. Clindamycin is also associated with *C. difficile* colitis, but in another way: a higher percentage of patients taking this over other antibiotics develop antibiotic-associated enterocolitis.

**64. The answer is b.** *(DiPalma, 4/e, p 738. Hardman and Limbird, 9/e, p 1062.)* Sulfonamides should not be used in pregnant women at term because of their ability to cross the placenta and enter the fetus in concentrations sufficient to produce toxic effects. Sulfonamides should also not be given to neonates, especially premature infants, because they compete with bilirubin for serum albumin binding, resulting in increased levels of free bilirubin, which causes kernicterus.

**65. The answer is a.** *(DiPalma, 4/e, pp 778–779. Hardman and Limbird, 9/e, pp 977–978.)* Primaquine is effective against the extraerythrocytic forms of *P. vivax* and *P. ovale* and is thus of value in a radical cure of malarial infection. It also attacks the sexual forms of the parasite, rendering them incapable of maturation in the mosquito and making it valuable in preventing the spread of malarial infection.

**66. The answer is b.** *(DiPalma, 4/e, pp 702–703. Hardman and Limbird, 9/e, p 1077.)* Unlike the other listed drugs, oxacillin is resistant to penicillinase. The other four agents are broad-spectrum penicillins, while oxacillin is generally specific for Gram-positive microorganisms. Use of penicillinase-resistant penicillins should be reserved for infections caused by penicillinase-producing staphylococci.

**67. The answer is e.** *(Hardman and Limbird, 9/e, p 1206. Katzung, 7/e, p 796.)* A major adverse effect of zidovudine is bone marrow depression that appears to be dose- and duration-dependent. The severity of the disease and a low CD4 count contribute to the bone marrow depression.

**68. The answer is c.** *(DiPalma, 4/e, pp 795–796. Hardman and Limbird, 9/e, p 1688.)* Thiabendazole (Mintezol) has been shown to be effective against *Strongyloides*, cutaneous larva migrans, and *Trichuris*. Adverse effects consist of nausea, vertigo, headache, and weakness. Treatment usually involves oral administration for several days. It has been found to be ineffective in *Ascaris*, *N. americanus*, *E. vermicularis*, and *T. saginata*.

(concluding)

**69. The answer is b.** (*Hardman and Limbird, 9/e, p 1299. Katzung, 7/e, p 925.*) Nephrotoxicity may occur in almost three-quarters of patients treated with cyclosporine. Regular monitoring of blood levels can reduce the incidence of adverse effects.

**70. The answer is c.** (*DiPalma, 4/e, pp 772–773. Hardman and Limbird, 9/e, pp 970–972.*) Chloroquine is a 4-aminoquinoline derivative that selectively concentrates in parasitized red blood cells. It is a weak base, and its alkalinizing effect on the acid vesicle of the parasite effectively destroys the viability of the parasite.

**71. The answer is c.** (*DiPalma, 4/e, p 742. Hardman and Limbird, 9/e, pp 1134–1135.*) Hematologic toxicity is by far the most important adverse effect of chloramphenicol. The toxicity consists of two types: bone marrow depression (common) and aplastic anemia (rare). Chloramphenicol can produce a potentially fatal toxic reaction, the gray baby syndrome, caused by diminished ability of neonates to conjugate chloramphenicol with resultant high serum concentrations. Tetracyclines produce staining of the teeth and phototoxicity.

**72. The answer is d.** (*DiPalma, 4/e, p 772. Hardman and Limbird, 9/e, p 989.*) Both trimethoprim-sulfamethoxazole and pentamidine are effective in pneumonia caused by *P. carinii*. This protozoal disease usually occurs in immunodeficient patients such as those with AIDS. Nifurtimox is effective in trypanosomiasis and metronidazole in amebiasis and leishmaniasis, as well as in anaerobic bacterial infections. Penicillins are not considered drugs of choice for this particular disease state.

**73. The answer is d.** (*Hardman and Limbird, 9/e, pp 1065–1067. Katzung, 7/e, p 765.*) Bacterial DNA gyrase is composed of four subunits, and norfloxacin binds to the strand-cutting subunits, inhibiting their activity.

**74. The answer is c.** (*Hardman and Limbird, 9/e, pp 1058–1059. Katzung, 7/e, pp 761–763.*) Trimethoprim inhibits dihydrofolic acid reductase. Sulfamethoxazole inhibits p-aminobenzoic acid (PABA) from being incorporated into folic acid by competitive inhibition of dihydropteroate synthase. Either action inhibits the synthesis of tetrahydrofolic acid.

**75. The answer is a.** (*Hardman and Limbird, 9/e, p 1157. Katzung, 7/e, p 771.*) INH inhibits mycobacterial cell wall synthesis by inhibiting mycolic acid synthesis by a mechanism that is not fully understood.

**76. The answer is a.** (*DiPalma, 4/e, p 176. Hardman and Limbird, 9/e, pp 1112–1113.*) Streptomycin, colistin, lincomycin, and clindamycin–in addition to neomycin listed in the question–have also been demonstrated to exert neuromuscular blocking effects that are synergistic with competitive blocking agents such as ether or tubocurarine. This effect is of clinical importance when these antibiotics are administered in large IV doses or intraperitoneally (IP).

**77. The answer is a.** (*DiPalma, 4/e, p 742. Hardman and Limbird, 9/e, p 1133.*) Chloramphenicol is the drug of choice in symptomatic *Salmonella* infection (typhoid fever) and also in *H. influenzae* meningitis in small children, especially when the strain is resistant to ampicillin. Tetracyclines are the drugs of choice for the treatment of brucellosis and cholera. Chloramphenicol may be used in the treatment of brucellosis, however, if tetracycline is contraindicated. Ordinary UTI and pharyngitis should be treated initially with penicillin.

**78. The answer is e.** (*Katzung, 7/e, pp 1064–1065.*) Cimetidine decreases the GI absorption of ketoconazole by lowering intestinal pH.

**79. The answer is a.** (*DiPalma, 4/e, pp 722–723. Hardman and Limbird, 9/e, pp 1110–1111.*) All the aminoglycosides are potentially toxic to both branches of the eighth cranial nerve. The evidence indicates that the sensory receptor portions of the inner ear are affected rather than the nerve itself. Nephrotoxicity may develop during or after the use of an aminoglycoside. It is generally more common in the elderly when there is preexisting renal dysfunction. In most patients renal function gradually improves after discontinuation of therapy. Aminoglycosides rarely cause neuromuscular blockade that can lead to progressive flaccid paralysis and potential fatal respiratory arrest. Hypersensitivity and dermatologic reactions occasionally occur following use of aminoglycosides.

**80. The answer is d.** (*Hardman and Limbird, 9/e, p 1200. Katzung, 7/e, p 794.*) Nephrotoxicity and symptomatic hypocalcemia are major toxicities associated with foscarnet. Underlying renal disease, concomitant use of nephrotoxic drugs, dehydration, and rapid infusion of high doses increase the risk.

**81. The answer is c.** *(Katzung, 7/e, p 797.)* Dideoxycytidine causes dose-dependent peripheral neuropathies and adverse effects in the GI tract, including nausea, diarrhea, and gastric and esophageal ulcerations and pancreatitis.

**82. The answer is b.** *(DiPalma, 4/e, pp 740–741. Hardman and Limbird, 9/e, p 1131.)* Chloramphenicol inhibits protein synthesis in bacteria and, to a lesser extent, in eukaryotic cells. The drug binds reversibly to the 50S ribosomal subunit and prevents attachment of aminoacyl-transfer RNA (tRNA) to its binding site. The amino acid substrate is unavailable for peptidyl transferase and peptide bond formation.

**83. The answer is d.** *(DiPalma, 4/e, pp 788, 792–793. Hardman and Limbird, 9/e, p 1019.)* Niclosamide is a halogenated salicylanilide derivative. It exerts its effect against cestodes by inhibition of mitochondrial oxidative phosphorylation in the parasites. The mechanism of action is also related to its inhibition of glucose and oxygen uptake in the parasite.

**84. The answer is a.** *(DiPalma, 4/e, pp 793–794. Hardman and Limbird, 9/e, pp 1020–1022.)* Praziquantel is a broad-spectrum antihelminthic agent. It appears to kill the adult schistosome by increasing the permeability of the cell membranes of the parasite to Ca and consequent influx of Ca ions. This causes increased muscle contraction followed by paralysis.

**85. The answer is a.** *(DiPalma, 4/e, pp 703–704. Hardman and Limbird, 9/e, pp 1084–1085.)* Amoxicillin is classified as an aminopenicillin along with ampicillin. Because it is less affected than ampicillin by the presence of food, it has a superior absorption in the GI tract. It is sensitive to penicillinase and has a narrow spectrum of activity toward certain Gram-positive and Gram-negative organisms, but not *Pseudomonas*. Since it is in the penicillin family, hypersensitivity reactions are a possibility.

**86. The answer is d.** *(DiPalma, 4/e, pp 693–695. Hardman and Limbird, 9/e, pp 1065–1068.)* β-Lactam antibiotics include penicillins, cephalosporins, monobactams, and carbapenems. All have a four-membered β-lactam ring that is essential for their antibacterial activity. Quinolones are fluorinated derivatives with no relationship chemically to the β-lactam antibiotics.

**87. The answer is e.** (*DiPalma, 4/e, pp 757–759. Hardman and Limbird, 9/e, pp 1178–1179.*) Amphotericin B disturbs the permeability and transport mechanisms of membranes by binding to ergosterol in the membrane. It is poorly absorbed via the oral route and must be given parenterally for the treatment of systemic fungal infections. In therapeutic concentrations, amphotericin B has the potential of causing both renal and liver damage, and the dose must be reduced when these toxicities develop. It has little or no activity in cell-wall synthesis.

**88. The answer is e.** (*DiPalma, 4/e, pp 693–694. Hardman and Limbird, 9/e, pp 1143–1144.*) Bacitracin, cycloserine, cephalothin, and vancomycin inhibit cell-wall synthesis and produce bacteria susceptible to environmental conditions. Polymyxins disrupt the structural integrity of the cytoplasmic membranes by acting as cationic detergents. On contact with the drug, the permeability of the membrane changes.

**89. The answer is c.** (*DiPalma, 4/e, pp 702–704. Hardman and Limbird, 9/e, p 1086.*) Ticarcillin resembles carbenicillin and has a high degree of potency against *Pseudomonas* and *Proteus* organisms but is broken down by penicillinase produced by various bacteria, including most staphylococci. Oxacillin, cloxacillin, nafcillin, and dicloxacillin are all resistant to penicillinase and are effective against staphylococci.

**90. The answer is e.** (*DiPalma, 4/e, pp 776–777. Hardman and Limbird, 9/e, pp 978–981.*) Quinine has analgesic and antipyretic properties similar to those of the salicylates. When applied locally, quinine has a local anesthetic action in which it briefly stimulates and then paralyzes sensory neurons. Because of its nature as protoplasmic poison, local destruction of tissue often results, which prolongs its action for weeks or months. When administered IV, quinine causes hypotension similar to that of its isomer quinidine.

**91. The answer is e.** (*DiPalma, 4/e, pp 764–765. Hardman and Limbird, 9/e, p 1202.*) Idoxuridine is a halogenated derivative of deoxyuridine. Its major action is on the DNA viruses, with little or no effect on RNA viruses. Its major use is in the treatment of herpes simplex keratitis, where it is usually used topically on the eye. When used topically, it may cause local irritation, photophobia, and occlusion of the lacrimal duct. Although effective against herpes simplex keratitis, idoxuridine is unresponsive to other herpes infections, including herpes simplex virus type 2 and varicella-zoster virus.

**92. The answer is e.** (*DiPalma, 4/e, pp 699–670. Hardman and Limbird, 9/e, pp 1086–1089.*) Allergic reactions are the main adverse effects encountered with the use of the penicillins. Sensitization is usually the result of previous treatment with a penicillin. Penicillins are not nephrotoxic; however, allergic interstitial nephritis may occur, particularly with methicillin. Hematologic reactions caused by penicillins are rare, but high concentrations may impair platelet function, resulting in prolongation of bleeding time. Seizures may develop when high doses of penicillins are given in the presence of renal insufficiency. Intolerance of alcohol (disulfiram-like reaction) has been noted only with certain cephalosporins.

**93. The answer is d.** (*DiPalma, 4/e, pp 706–714. Hardman and Limbird, 9/e, pp 1074–1077.*) Cephalosporins and penicillins have similar structures, penicillins having a penicillic acid and the cephalosporins a cephalosporinic acid moiety. Both groups of antimicrobials inhibit the transpeptidase enzyme necessary for cross-linking. It appears that the mechanism is not totally identical for every drug for every bacterial species. Cephalosporins have a greater overall activity against Gram-negative organisms than do the penicillin G-type compounds. The hypersensitivity reactions associated with the penicillins and the cephalosporins appear to be identical in signs and symptoms. There is a cross-over sensitivity between the penicillins and cephalosporins that must be considered when a patient is sensitive to either of these antibiotics.

**94. The answer is b.** (*DiPalma, 4/e, pp 702–703. Hardman and Limbird, 9/e, p 1077.*) Methicillin is classified as a penicillinase-resistant penicillin that is acid-labile and therefore not useful for oral administration. Major adverse reactions include penicillin hypersensitivity and interstitial nephritis. With the exception of methicillin, which is 35% bound to serum proteins, all penicillinase-resistant penicillins are highly bound to plasma proteins.

**95. The answer is e.** (*DiPalma, 4/e, pp 735–736. Hardman and Limbird, 9/e, pp 995–998.*) Metronidazole is a low-molecular-weight compound that penetrates all tissues and fluids of the body. Metronidazole's spectrum of activity is limited largely to anaerobic bacteria—including *B. fragilis*—and certain protozoa. It is considered to be the drug of choice for trichomoniasis in females and carrier states in males as well as intestinal infections with *Giardia lamblia*.

**96. The answer is e.** (*DiPalma, 4/e, pp 707–708. Hardman and Limbird, 9/e, p 1093.*) In about 5% of the patients receiving cephalothin, a hypersensitivity reaction develops that is characterized by fever, eosinophilia, serum sickness, rash, and anaphylaxis. A positive Coombs' test result is also frequent but is seldom associated with hemolytic anemia. Thrombophlebitis with IV administration of cephalothin is almost universal. Superinfection by cephalothin-resistant Gram-negative bacilli has been noted by several observers. The cephalosporins have also been implicated as potentially nephrotoxic agents.

**97. The answer is e.** (*DiPalma, 4/e, pp 763–764. Hardman and Limbird, 9/e, pp 1195–1198.*) Acyclovir is a nucleoside analogue of the pyrimidine guanosine. The mechanism of activity involves its conversion to a triphosphate and subsequent inhibition of synthesis of viral DNA. Its activity is highly selective. Acyclovir is available for topical, oral, and IV administration and is highly effective against herpes simplex, varicella-zoster, and Epstein-Barr viruses.

**98. The answer is a.** (*DiPalma, 4/e, pp 704–705. Hardman and Limbird, 9/e, p 1086.*) Carbenicillin has a carboxyl group on the side chain and thus is not an aminopenicillin. It is classified as an extended-spectrum penicillin with a wide range of activity against anaerobic Gram-negative organisms. It is susceptible to staphylococcal penicillinase organisms. When given with aminoglycosides, a synergistic activity will occur against many isolates of *P. aeruginosa.*

**99. The answer is d.** (*DiPalma, 4/e, pp 744–745. Hardman and Limbird, 9/e, p 1127.*) Tetracyclines, as chelating agents, have a high affinity for the divalent cations of Ca and Mg salts, as well as for iron (Fe)-containing preparations, dairy products, and aluminum hydroxide [$Al(OH)_3$] gels. The chelated complex is insoluble and not absorbed through the GI tract mucosa. Tetracyclines should be administered before meals to prevent formation of such chelates. Antacids that contain cations of Ca, Mg, or Al should not be administered simultaneously with tetracyclines.

**100–102. The answers are 100-c, 101-g, 102-a.** (*DiPalma, 4/e, pp 788–790. Katzung, 7/e, pp 865–867, 876.*) Pinworm infestation should be treated with pyrantel in conjunction with rigid standards of personal hygiene. Pyrantel is also the drug of choice against *A. lumbricoides.* A single dose of 11 mg/kg, to a maximum of 1 g, is sufficient.

Filariasis is effectively treated with diethylcarbamazine, a piperazine derivative, which both suppresses and, in most cases, cures the infection. The drug is inactive against *W. bancrofti* in vitro. However, in vivo activity appears to be due to a sensitization of the microfilaria to phagocytosis by the fixed macrophages of the reticuloendothelial system.

Bithionol has been found useful in the treatment of infection by the sheep liver fluke *F. hepatica* and the lung fluke *Paragonimus kellicotti*. Treatment usually involves the oral administration of 40 to 50 mg/kg, in divided doses on alternate days, for a total of 10 to 15 doses. Chloroquine in large doses has also been successful in the therapy of infection by lung flukes.

**103–105. The answers are 103-f, 104-a, 105-c.** *(DiPalma, 4/e, pp 700–705. Katzung, 7/e, pp 728–732.)* Because of its long duration of action, benzathine penicillin G is given as a single injection of 1.2 million units IM every 3 or 4 weeks for the treatment of syphilis. This persistence of action reduces the need for repeated injections, costs, and local trauma. Benzathine penicillin G is also administered for group A, β-hemolytic streptococcal pharyngitis and pyoderma.

Methicillin is a β-lactamase-resistant (penicillinase-resistant) penicillin that is acid-labile but must be administered by the parenteral route. It is effective against nearly all strains of *S. aureus*. Methicillin is much more effective against penicillinase-producing strains than is penicillin G.

Piperacillin along with mezlocillin and azlocillin is commonly referred to as an extended-spectrum penicillin because of its broad spectrum of activity. It is particularly effective against *Klebsiella* and *Pseudomonas*. Piperacillin is available as a powder for solubilization and injection.

# CANCER CHEMOTHERAPY AND IMMUNOLOGY

**Note: In the classification of drugs, prototype drugs are marked with an asterisk (\*).**

The Cell Cycle
- Effect of various chemotherapeutic agents on different stages of the cell cycle
- General toxicities of chemotherapeutic agents on normal tissues

Alkylating Agents
- Nitrogen mustards
  - Mechlorethamine hydrochloride (HCl)*
  - Chlorambucil
  - Melphalan
  - Ifosfamide
  - Cyclophosphamide
  - Uracil mustard
- Nitrosoureas
  - Lomustine*
  - Carmustine
  - Streptozocin
- Miscellaneous
  - Thiotepa
  - Busulfan
  - Dacarbazine (DTIC)
  - Pipobroman
  - Procarbazine
  - Cisplatin*
  - Carboplatin

Antimetabolites
- Methotrexate, trimetrexate
- Mercaptopurine, thioguanine
- Fluorouracil (FU), floxuridine, fludarabine, cladribine, and pentostatin
- Cytarabine

Hormones
- Androgens
  - Testolactone*
- Antiandrogen
  - Flutamide*
- Glucocorticosteroids
  - Prednisone
  - Prednisolone
- Progestins
  - Megestrol acetate*
  - Medroxyprogesterone acetate
- Estrogens
  - Diethylstilbestrol diphosphate*
  - Polyestradiol phosphate
- Estrogen/nitrogen mustard
  - Estramustine phosphate sodium
- Antiestrogen
  - Tamoxifen citrate*
- Gonadotropin-releasing hormone analogue

**57**

Leuprolide acetate*
Goserelin acetate
Antibiotics
Bleomycin sulfate*
Anthracyclines
Idarubicin HCl
Doxorubicin HCl*
Daunorubicin HCl
Mitoxantrone HCl
Mitomycin*
Dactinomycin
Plicamycin
Plant derivatives
Etoposide
Teniposide
Vincristine sulfate*
Vinblastine sulfate
Paclitaxel
Miscellaneous
Interferon α-2a, α-2b, α-n3*
Levamisole HCl*
Altretamine
Hydroxyurea
Bacille bilié de Calmette-Guérin (BCG) intravesical
Mitotane
Asparaginase*
Radiopharmaceuticals
Sodium iodide (NaI) $^{131}I$*
Sodium phosphate $^{32}P$
Immunopharmacologic Drugs
Cytotoxic
Azathioprine*
Cyclophosphamide
Vincristine
Methotrexate
Cytarabine
Specific T-cell inhibitor
Cyclosporine*
Hormonal
Prednisone*
Other corticosteroids
Antibodies
Antilymphocyte globulin (ALG)
Muromonab-$CD_3$
$Rh_o$(D) immune globulin

Melphalan ? Busulphan ] alkylating
Bleomycin - Antibiotic
Dacarbazine ] Alkylating
Procarbazine
Daunorubicin ] Antibiotics
Doxorubicin

# Questions

**DIRECTIONS:** Each question below contains several suggested responses. Select the **one best** response to each question.

**106.** The most effective drug for immunosuppression of rejection of the allografted kidney is

a. azathioprine
b. cyclosporine
c. 5-FU
d. cyclophosphamide
e. vincristine

**107.** The phase of the cell cycle that is resistant to most chemotherapeutic agents and requires increased dosage to obtain a response is

a. M phase
b. $G_2$ phase
c. S phase
d. $G_0$ phase
e. $G_1$ phase

**108.** A nucleophilic attack on deoxyribonucleic acid (DNA) that causes the disruption of base pairing occurs as a result of administration of

a. cyclophosphamide
b. 5-FU
c. methotrexate
d. prednisone
e. thioguanine

**109.** The antineoplastic chemotherapeutic agent that is classified as an alkylating agent is

a. thioguanine
b. busulfan
c. bleomycin
d. vincristine
e. tamoxifen

**110.** Which of the following is a chemotherapeutic drug that possesses a mechanism of action involving alkylation?

a. cyclophosphamide
b. methotrexate
c. tamoxifen
d. 5-FU
e. bleomycin

**111.** A nine-year-old boy is diagnosed with acute lymphoblastic leukemia. He is maintained on methotrexate. A recent platelet count is below normal, and a stool guaiac is 4+. Which of the following agents should be administered to counteract methotrexate toxicity?

a. N-acetylcysteine
b. vitamin K
c. penicillamine
d. leucovorin
e. deferoxamine

**112.** Cardiotoxicity limits the clinical usefulness of which one of the following antitumor antibiotics?

a. dactinomycin
b. doxorubicin
c. bleomycin
d. cisplatin
e. vincristine

**113.** Binding to the enzyme dihydrofolate reductase is the mechanism of action for

a. procarbazine
b. paclitaxel
c. methotrexate
d. ifosfamide
e. cladribine

**114.** Which of the following is considered to be the effective mechanism of action of the vinca alkaloids?

a. inhibition of the function of microtubules
b. damage and prevention of repair of DNA
c. inhibition of DNA synthesis
d. inhibition of protein synthesis
e. inhibition of purine synthesis

**DIRECTIONS:** Each numbered question or incomplete statement below is NEGATIVELY phrased. Select the **one best** lettered response.

**115.** The tumor LEAST susceptible to cell cycle-specific (CCS) anticancer agents is

a. acute lymphoblastic leukemia
b. acute granulocytic leukemia
c. Burkitt's lymphoma
d. adenocarcinoma of the colon
e. choriocarcinoma

**116.** A 32-year-old cancer patient, who has smoked two packs of cigarettes a day for 10 years, presents a decreased pulmonary function test. Physical examination and chest x-rays suggest preexisting pulmonary disease. All the following drugs may be prescribed EXCEPT

a. vinblastine
b. doxorubicin
c. mithramycin
d. bleomycin
e. cisplatin

**117.** All the following are CCS agents EXCEPT

a. mercaptopurine (6-MP)
b. 5-FU
c. bleomycin
d. busulfan
e. vincristine

**118.** All the following statements regarding the chemotherapy of cancer are valid EXCEPT

a. 50% of all newly diagnosed cancer patients will be cured of their disease
b. chemotherapy is the only treatment that can effectively treat systemic disease
c. chemotherapy only kills cancer cells and not normal dividing cells
d. chemotherapy possesses numerous side effects, such as nausea, vomiting, and suppression of bone marrow

**119.** Paclitaxel, an agent extracted from the yew tree, has all the following actions and uses EXCEPT

a. it promotes premature cell division
b. it can cause neutropenia
c. it causes disorganized microtubule bundles
d. it is used to treat metastatic breast cancer
e. it is a competitive inhibitor at the estrogen receptor

**120.** Alkylating agents perhaps the most useful agents in cancer chemotherapy, have all the following actions EXCEPT

a. they are able to form covalent bonds with nucleophilic sites on nucleic acids
b. they possess little or no toxicity in the host
c. they are cytotoxic owing to their activity against DNA
d. they are able to form a positive carbonium ion
e. they can affect any part of the cell cycle

**121.** A 34-year-old male with Hodgkin's disease is treated with the adriamycin, bleomycin, vinblastine, and decarbazine (ABVD) regimen. What is vinblastine's mechanism of action?

a. scission of DNA strands
b. inhibition of dihydrofolate reductase
c. inhibition of enzymes involved in purine metabolism
d. prevention of assembly of tubulin dimers into microtubules
e. inhibition of topoisomerase

**122.** Drugs classified as immuno-stimulants include all the following EXCEPT

a. interferon $\alpha$
b. aldesleukin $-23$ $(IL-2)$
c. muromonab-CD3
d. sargramostim $\Big\}$ CSF
e. filgrastim

**123.** Levamisole is an unusual cancer chemotherapeutic agent. It has all the following attributes EXCEPT

a. antihelminthic properties
b. immunostimulation
c. effectiveness in colon cancer with 5-FU
d. metallic taste
e. inhibition of monocyte chemotaxis

**DIRECTIONS:** Each group of questions below consists of lettered headings followed by a set of numbered items. For each numbered item select the **one** lettered heading with which it is **most** closely associated. Each lettered heading may be used **once, more than once, or not at all.**

## Questions 124–126

For each of the drugs below, select the characteristic with which it is most likely to be associated.

a.  used in treatment of Hodgkin's lymphoma
b.  classified as an alkylating agent and orally administered
c.  retained specifically in β cells of the islets of Langerhans
d.  used as a single agent against malignant melanoma
e.  classified as an antitumor antibiotic and results in a high incidence of bone marrow suppression
f.  used in treatment of breast cancer
g.  classified as a vinca alkaloid
h.  used in malignant hypercalcemia
i.  used in hairy cell leukemia
j.  derived from hydrazine

*C* **124.** Streptozocin

*d* **125.** DTIC (Mal. Melanoma)

*e* **126.** Mitomycin    Antis Tumour biotin

## Questions 127–129

For each of the indications below, select the correct drug.

a.  allopurinol
b.  asparaginase
c.  methotrexate
d.  streptozocin
e.  6-MP
f.  azathioprine
g.  pentostatin
h.  leucovorin
i.  BCG vaccine

*c* **127.** Severe active rheumatoid arthritis    Metho.

*f* **128** Renal allografts    Azathro.

*i* **129.** Bladder cancer    BCG.

**Questions 130–132**

For each of the drugs below, select the adverse reaction with which it is most closely associated.

a. aseptic hemorrhagic cystitis
b. cardiotoxicity
c. nephrotoxicity
d. oral and gastrointestinal (GI) ulceration
e. exfoliative dermatitis
f. peripheral neuropathy
g. convulsions
h. pancreatitis
i. coma

**130.** 5-FU    *(c i t)*

**131.** Asparaginase    *Pancreatitis*

**132.** Procarbazine    *(for Neuropathy)*

---

**Questions 133–135**

For each of the chemotherapeutic agents below, choose the phase of the cell cycle at which it is most likely to act.

**133.** Busulfan

**134.** Dactinomycin

**135.** DTIC

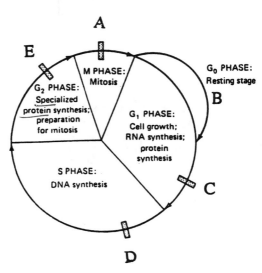

# CANCER CHEMOTHERAPY AND IMMUNOLOGY

## Answers

**106. The answer is b.** *(DiPalma, 4/e, pp 681–683. Hardman and Limbird, 9/e, pp 1296–1299.)* Cyclosporine is the preferred agent because it is a specific T-cell inhibitor and its success rate in protecting against rejection is considerably better than that of any other agent. All the other agents listed in the question are cytotoxic. Because of the severe adverse reactions with cyclosporine, it is used in conjunction with azathioprine, which reduces the required dose. Prednisone is also used in conjunction with cyclosporine.

**107. The answer is d.** *(AMA Drug Evaluations Annual, 1993, p 1938. DiPalma, 4/e, pp 653–655.)* There are various phases described for the cell cycle. The M phase is the period of cell division (mitosis). Following the M phase a cell may enter either the $G_1$ phase or $G_0$ phase. The $G_1$ phase of the cell cycle is associated with cell growth, ribonucleic acid (RNA) synthesis, and protein synthesis. The $G_0$ phase is the resting or dormant stage. No cell division takes place, although the cells are still capable of undergoing mitosis. This phase of the cell cycle is the most resistant to chemotherapeutic agents and may require a high dosage of the chemotherapeutic agent because most cancer drugs produce their lethal effect on cells that are actively involved in division. The S phase of the cell cycle involves DNA synthesis, and cells that are in the $G_2$ phase show the synthesis of specialized proteins in preparation for cell replication.

**108. The answer is a.** *(DiPalma, 4/e, pp 665–666. Hardman and Limbird, 9/e, p 1302.)* Cyclophosphamide, an alkylating agent, reacts with purine and pyrimidine bases of DNA to form bridges and dimers. These products interfere with DNA replication. 5-FU, methotrexate, and 6-thioguanine are antimetabolites, and the steroid prednisone has some tumor-suppressive effects.

**109. The answer is b.** *(DiPalma, 4/e, p 657. Hardman and Limbird, 9/e, p 1241.)* Busulfan is an alkylating agent that, in contrast to other alkylators, is an alkylsulfonate. Thioguanine is a purine antimetabolite. Bleomycin is classified as a chemotherapeutic antibiotic and vincristine is a vinca alkaloid. Tamoxifen is an antiestrogen hormone.

**110. The answer is a.** (*DiPalma, 4/e, p 657. Hardman and Limbird, 9/e, p 1302.*) Cyclophosphamide is classified as a polyfunctional alkylating drug that transfers its alkyl groups to cellular components. The cytotoxic effect of this agent is directly associated with the alkylation of components of DNA. Methotrexate and FU are classified as antimetabolites that block intermediary metabolism to inhibit cell proliferation. Tamoxifen is an antiestrogen compound. Bleomycin is classified as an antibiotic chemotherapeutic agent.

**111. The answer is d.** (*Hardman and Limbird, 9/e, pp 1247, 1335.*) Leucovorin prevents methotrexate from inhibiting dihydrofolate reductase and reverses all of its adverse effects except neurotoxicity.

**112. The answer is b.** (*DiPalma, 4/e, pp 667–669. Hardman and Limbird, 9/e, pp 1264–1265.*) Dactinomycin's major toxicities include stomatitis, alopecia, and bone marrow depression. Bleomycin's toxicities include edema of the hands, alopecia, and stomatitis. Cisplatin produces both nephrotoxicity and ototoxicity. The clinical toxicity of vincristine is mostly neurologic. Doxorubicin causes cardiotoxicity as well as alopecia and bone marrow depression. The cardiotoxicity has been linked to a lipid peroxidation within cardiac cells.

**113. The answer is c.** (*AMA Drug Evaluations Annual, 1994, p 1990. DiPalma, 4/e, p 656. Hardman and Limbird, 9/e, pp 1243–1247.*) Antimetabolites of folic acid such as methotrexate, which is an important cancer chemotherapeutic agent, exert their effect by inhibiting the catalytic activity of the enzyme dihydrofolate reductase. The enzyme functions to keep folic acid in a reduced state. The first step in the reaction is the reduction of folic acid to 7,8-dihydrofolic acid ($FH_2$), which requires the cofactor nicotinic acid adenine dinucleotide phosphate (NADPH). The second step is the conversion of $FH_2$ to 5,6,7,8-tetrahydrofolic acid ($FH_4$). This part of the reduction reaction requires nicotinic acid adenine dinucleotide (NADH) or NADPH. The reduced forms of folic acid are involved in one-carbon transfer reactions that are required during the synthesis of purines and pyrimidine thymidylate. The affinity of methotrexate for dihydrofolate reductase is much greater than for the substrates of folic acid and dihydrofolic acid. The action of methotrexate can be blocked or reduced by the administration of leucovorin ($N^5$-formyl $FH_4$), which can substitute for the reduced forms of folic acid in the cell. Methotrexate affects the S phase of the cell cycle. The drug is actively transported into the cell and at very large doses the drug can enter the cell by simple diffusion. Although cladribine is an antimetabolite, it does not inhibit dihydrofolate reductase. Procarbazine, paclitaxel, and ifosfamide exert their anticancer effects through other mechanisms of action that are not associated with dihydrofolate reductase.

**114. The answer is a.** (*DiPalma, 4/e, p 671. Hardman and Limbird, 9/e, pp 1259, 1260.*) The vinca alkaloids vincristine and vinblastine have proved valuable because they work on a different principle from most cancer chemotherapeutic agents. They (like colchicine) inhibit mitosis in metaphase by their ability to bind to tubulin. This prevents the formation of tubules and consequently the orderly arrangement of chromosomes, which apparently causes cell death.

**115. The answer is d.** (*DiPalma, 4/e, pp 653-656.*) CCS cytotoxic agents are most effective in malignancies in which a large portion of the population of malignant cells is undergoing mitosis. In leukemia, lymphoma, choriocarcinoma, and other rapidly growing tumors, these agents may induce a high-percentage cell kill of the entire tumor and at least of those cells that are actively dividing. In slowly growing, solid tumors, such as carcinomas of the colon, the frequency of actively dividing cells is low, and perhaps the resting cells survive the cycle-specific agents and then can be recruited back into the proliferative cycle.

**116. The answer is d.** (*AMA Drug Evaluations Annual, 1993, pp 1174–1175. DiPalma, 4/e, pp 668–669.*) The potential serious adverse effect of bleomycin is pneumonitis and pulmonary fibrosis. This adverse effect appears to be both age and dose-related. The clinical onset is characterized by decreasing pulmonary function, fine rales, cough, and diffuse basilar infiltrates. This complication develops in approximately 5% to 10% of patients treated with bleomycin. Thus, extreme caution must be used in patients with a preexisting history of pulmonary disease. All the other drugs listed in the question are effective against carcinomas and have not been associated with significant lung toxicity.

**117. The answer is d.** (*DiPalma, 4/e, pp 654–656. Hardman and Limbird, 9/e, p 1236.*) CCS agents such as 6-MP, FU, bleomycin, and vincristine have proved to be the most effective against proliferating cells. Busulfan is an alkylating agent that binds to DNA and causes damage to these macromolecules. It is useful against low-growth as well as high-growth tumors and is classified as a cell cycle-nonspecific (CCNS) agent.

**118. The answer is c.** (*DiPalma, 4/e, pp 653–656. Katzung, 7/e, pp 881–884.*) Cancer chemotherapy, even with the best and most efficient detection procedures, can cure only approximately 50% of all newly diagnosed cancer patients. The reason for failure to cure is not delay in diagnosis. Surgery, chemotherapy, and radiation constitute the three forms of treatment for cancer, but only chemotherapy can effectively treat systemic disease. Both normal and cancerous dividing cells are killed by chemotherapy, which is one of its major drawbacks. Other serious side effects include nausea, vomiting, and suppression of bone marrow. The newer agents are specifically designed for their specific effects on the cell cycle.

**119. The answer is e.** (*DiPalma, 4/e, pp 672–673. Hardman and Limbird, 9/e, pp 1260–1262.*) Paclitaxel is a large structural molecule that contains a 15-membered taxane ring system. This anticancer agent is derived from the bark of the Pacific yew tree. Its chemotherapeutic action is related to the microtubules in the cell. Paclitaxel promotes microtubule assembly from dimers and causes microtubule stabilization by preventing depolymerization. As a consequence of these actions, the microtubules form disorganized bundles, which decreases interphase and mitotic function. Furthermore, paclitaxel also causes premature cell division. The drug is administered intravenously and is useful in such diseases as cisplatin-resistant ovarian cancer, metastatic breast cancer, malignant melanoma, and acute myelogenous leukemia. Adverse reactions reported from the use of paclitaxel include dose-dependent neutropenia, hypersensitivity reactions, mild neuropathy, transient myalgias and arthralgias, and rarely bradyarrhythmias. The cancer therapeutic agent that competitively inhibits the binding of estradiol to estrogen receptors is the oral antiestrogen tamoxifen, which is employed in the treatment of receptor-positive postmenopausal women with breast cancer.

**120. The answer is b.** (*DiPalma, 4/e, pp 663–664. Hardman and Limbird, 9/e, pp 1236–1238.*) The alkylating agents are highly reactive compounds with the ability to form covalent bonds with nucleophilic sites on molecules such as nucleic acids. This is usually accomplished through the formation of a positively charged carbonium ion. The cytotoxic effects of these agents most likely reflect their ability to bind to the nucleotides of DNA. The alkylators have an effect during any part of the cell cycle (CCNS). Because of their nonspecificity, these compounds produce a significant number of adverse effects in the host.

**121. The answer is d.** *(Hardman and Limbird, 9/e, p 1258. Katzung, 7/e, p 893.)* Vinblastine binds to tubulin and blocks the protein from polymerizing to microtubules. The drug-tubulin complex binds to the developing microtubule, resulting in inhibition of microtubule assembly and subsequent depolymerization.

**122. The answer is c.** *(DiPalma, 4/e, pp 677–680, 684–687. Hardman and Limbird, 9/e, p 1302.)* Muromonab-CD3 is a monoclonal antibody that interferes with T-cell function. It is classified as an immunosuppressive drug. This drug is given intravenously and is indicated in the treatment of acute allograft rejection. Generally, azathioprine and prednisone are used along with muromonab-CD3. Interferon α and aldesleukin (interleukin-2) are cytokines that are classified as immunostimulants. Sargramostim and filgrastim are also immunostimulants. These drugs are produced by recombinant DNA technology. Sargramostim is a human granulocyte macrophage colony stimulating factor (GM-CSF) and filgrastim is a human granulocyte colony stimulating factor (G-CSF).

**123. The answer is e.** *(DiPalma, 4/e, pp 678, 687. Hardman and Limbird, 9/e, p 1291.)* Levamisole was used as an antihelminthic agent. It is now indicated in the therapy of advanced colon cancer in combination with 5-FU. Levamisole is classified as an immunostimulant; however, this action is dose-dependent and related to duration of administration. Its main effect may be due to enhancement of monocyte chemotaxis; however, it also causes increased monocyte phagocytosis and increased activity of neutrophils. Levamisole produces adverse reactions such as flulike symptoms, nausea, vomiting, blurred vision, convulsions, and a metallic taste. In addition, the drug may cause an alteration in the sense of smell.

**124–126. The answers are 124-c, 125-d, 126-e.** *(DiPalma, 4/e, pp 666–669. Hardman and Limbird, 9/e, pp 1242–1243, 1269.)* Streptozocin is a nitrosourea-like antibiotic that contains a glucosamine moiety that allows it to be selectively taken up by the beta cells of the islets of Langerhans. Consequently, it appears to be useful in treating metastatic islet cell carcinoma.

DTIC is a triazene derivative of alkylating agents that appears to require demethylation for activity. It has displayed significant anti-neoplastic action against malignant melanomas.

Mitomycin is a potent antibiotic that selectively inhibits DNA synthesis by its ability to alkylate and cross-link DNA. The drug causes a bone marrow suppression in up to 64% of patients.

**127–129. The answers are 127-c, 128-f, 129-i.** (*DiPalma, 4/e, pp 656–659, 661, 672, 677–681, 687–689.*) Methotrexate is classified as an antimetabolite with therapeutic uses in cancer chemotherapy and as an immunosuppressive agent indicated in the treatment of severe active classical rheumatoid arthritis. Leucovorin is related to methotrexate in that it is an antagonist of its actions. It can supply a source of reduced folate for the methylation reactions that are prevented by methotrexate.

Azathioprine is a derivative closely related to 6-MP, which is used as a cancer chemotherapeutic agent while azathioprine is used as an immunosuppressive agent because it is more effective than 6-MP in this regard. Azathioprine is used in organ transplantation, particularly kidney allografts. Like 6-MP, azathioprine is biotransformed to inactive product by xanthine oxidase. Allopurinol, which inhibits this enzyme, can increase the therapeutic action of azathioprine and possibly its adverse reactions. The dosage of azathioprine should be decreased in the presence of allopurinol.

BCG vaccine is a nonspecific stimulant of the reticuloendothelial system. It is an attenuated strain of *Mycobacterium bovis* that appears most effective in small, localized bladder tumors. This agent is approved for intravesicular use in bladder cancer. Adverse reactions are associated with the renal system, such as problems with urination, infection, and cystitis.

**130–132. The answers are 130-d, 131-h, 132-f.** (*DiPalma, 4/e, pp 662, 665–668, 672–673. Hardman and Limbird, 9/e, pp 1251–1252, 1270, 1272–1273.*) FU is a pyrimidine antagonist that has a low neurotoxicity when compared with other fluorinated derivatives; however, its major toxicities are myelosuppression and oral or gastrointestinal ulceration. Leukopenia is the most frequent clinical manifestation of the myelosuppression.

Asparaginase is an enzyme that catalyzes the hydrolysis of serum asparagine to aspartic acid and ammonia. Major toxicities are related to antigenicity and pancreatitis. In addition, more than 50% of those treated present biochemical evidence of hepatic dysfunction.

Procarbazine commonly produces a dose-related, reversible bone marrow depression including thrombocytopenia and leukopenia. Neurotoxicity is also associated with this drug in 10% to 20% of the patients receiving it. This is manifested as ataxia, disorders in consciousness, and peripheral neuropathies. Procarbazine may reduce plasma pyridoxal phosphate levels, a phenomenon that may be responsible for the neurotoxicity.

**133–135. The answers are 133-b, 134-d, 135-e.** (*DiPalma, 4/e, pp 653–656, 667–668.*) Specific cell-cycle events are present in both normal and cancerous cells. These phases of the cell cycle are shown in the diagram with the questions. Although general statements can be made regarding the cell-cycle phases in which certain classes of chemotherapeutic agents act, some drugs listed in a particular category of antineoplastic agents may exhibit their effects on a different phase of the cell cycle. Alkylating agents are considered to be nonspecific in regard to the phase at which they have their effects. However, the alkylating agents DTIC and busulfan are mostly active during the $G_2$ phase and the $G_0$ phase, respectively. In addition, antibiotic chemotherapeutic agents are considered to have effect in the $G_2$ phase of the cell cycle. The antibiotic agent dactinomycin, however, is most active in the S phase.

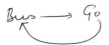

# CARDIOVASCULAR AND PULMONARY SYSTEMS

**Note: In the classification of drugs, prototype drugs are marked with an asterisk (\*).**

Cardiac Glycosides

Digoxin, digitoxin, deslanoside

Other Inotropic Agents

Sympathomimetics

Epinephrine,* isoproterenol,* dopamine,* dobutamine

Nonsympathomimetics

Theophylline,* amrinone,* milrinone

Vasodilators for Congestive Heart Failure

Nitrates, sodium nitroprusside, captopril, enalapril, lisinopril, quinapril, ramipril, nifedipine, nicardipine

Antiarrhythmic Drugs

1A. Quinidine,* procainamide, disopyramide

1B. Lidocaine,* tocainide, mexiletine, phenytoin

1C. Flecainide,* encainide, propafenone

2. Propranolol (other ( blockers)

3. Amiodarone,* bretylium, sotalol

4. Verapamil, diltiazem

5. Adenosine

Antianginal Drugs

Nitrates and nitrites

Nitroglycerine,* amyl nitrite, pentaerythritol tetranitrate, isosorbide dinitrate

β-adrenergic blocking drugs

(All members are useful; a good choice is the cardioselective ones such as acebutolol, atenolol, and metoprolol)

Calcium channel blockers

Nifedipine, verapamil, diltiazem, bepridil

Agents for hyperlipoproteinemia

Bile acid sequestrants

Colestipol, cholestyramine

Nicotinic acid (NA)

Clofibrate, gemfibrozil

Probucol

Lovastatin

Antihypertensive Drugs

Thiazides (benzothiadiazides)

(All are effective; most commonly used are chlorothiazide and hydrochlorothiazide—see section on Diuretics)

Sympatholytic agents

Centrally acting

Methyldopa, clonidine, guanabenz, guanfacine

Peripherally acting
β-adrenergic blocking agents
  Propranolol, etc.
α-adrenergic blocking
  agents
    Prazosin, terazosin,
    reserpine, guanethidine,
    guanadrel
Arterial vasodilators
  Hydralazine, minoxidil
Angiotensin-converting enzyme
  (ACE) inhibitors
    Captopril, enalapril, lisinopril,
    quinapril, fosinopril, ramipril
Calcium (Ca) channel-blockers
    Nifedipine, verapamil,
    diltiazem, amlodipine,
    nicardipine
Drugs for hypertensive
  emergencies
    Trimethaphan, sodium
    nitroprusside, diazoxide,
    nifedipine, labetalol
Drugs for Chronic Obstructive
  Pulmonary Disease (COPD)
Bronchodilators
  Methylxanthines, theophylline,
    elixophyllin
  β-receptor agonists
    Epinephrine, isoproterenol,
    isoetharine, metaproterenol,
    terbutaline, albuterol
  Anticholinergics
    Atropine, ipratropium*
  Mediator-release inhibitors
    Cromolyn sodium,*
    nedocromil

Corticosteroids
  Flunisolide, beclomethasone,
    triamcinolone
Mucokinetic agents
  Acetylcysteine
  Guaifenesin
  Iodide
  Saline
Hematologic Agents
Antianemia drugs
  Iron-ferrous sulfate, vitamin
    $B_{12}$, folic acid
  Iron (Fe) detoxifiers,
    deferoxamine
Anticoagulant and procoagulant
  drugs
  Parenteral anticoagulants
    Heparin and enoxaparin
  Oral anticoagulants
    Warfarin and dicumarol
  Inhibitors of platelet aggregation
    Aspirin and other nonsteroidal
    anti-inflammatory drugs
    (NSAIDs)
  Fibrinolytic drugs
    Streptokinase, tissue plas-
    minogen activator (tPA–
    alteplase), anistreplase
  Procoagulant drugs
    Systemic
    Antihemophilic factor, factor
    VIII, factor IX complex,
    desmopressin, aminocaproic
    acid, tranexamic acid
  Topical
    Thrombin, absorbable
    gelatin, oxidized cellulose

# Questions

**DIRECTIONS:** Each question below contains several suggested responses. Select the **one best** response to each question.

**136.** The cardiovascular responses of a normal man were recorded and are shown in the accompanying figure following a 15-min infusion of drug X. Which of the following was most likely drug X?

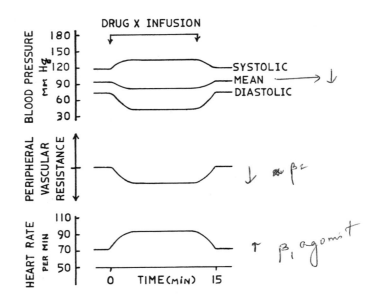

a. methacholine
b. propranolol
c. atropine
d. isoproterenol
e. norepinephrine

**137.** A 75-year-old female in CHF is unable to climb a flight of stairs without experiencing shortness of breath. Digoxin is administered to improve cardiac muscle contractility. Within two weeks, she has a marked improvement in her symptoms. What cellular action of digoxin accounts for this?

a. inhibition of cyclic adenosine monophosphate (AMP) synthesis
b. inhibition of mitochondrial Ca release
c. inhibition of the sodium (Na) pump
d. inhibition of β-adrenergic stimulation
e. inhibition of adenosine triphosphate (ATP) degradation

**138.** In a patient who has had attacks of paroxysmal atrial tachycardia, an ideal prophylactic drug is

a. adenosine
b. procainamide
c. lidocaine
d. nifedipine
e. verapamil

**139.** The therapeutic action of β-adrenergic receptor blockers such as propranolol in angina pectoris is believed to be primarily the result of

a. reduced production of catecholamines
b. dilation of the coronary vasculature
c. decreased requirement for myocardial oxygen
d. increased peripheral resistance
e. increased sensitivity to catecholamines

**140.** A 59-year-old female with mild CHF is treated with furosemide. What is its primary mechanism of action?

a. inhibition of sodium-potassium (Na⁺/K⁺) adenosine triphosphatase (ATPase)
b. inhibition of Na⁺/K⁺/chloride (Cl⁻) cotransporter
c. inhibition of Na⁺/Cl⁻ cotransporter
d. inhibition of Cl⁻ transporter
e. inhibition of Ca divalent cation (Ca⁺⁺) transporter

**141.** A positive Coombs' test and hemolytic anemia may follow the administration of which antihypertensive drug?

a. methyldopa
b. clonidine
c. guanabenz
d. prazosin
e. captopril

**142.** Which of the following is an antiarrhythmic agent that has relatively few electrophysiologic effects on normal myocardial tissue but suppresses the arrhythmogenic tendencies of ischemic myocardial tissues?

a. propranolol
b. procainamide
c. quinidine
d. lidocaine
e. disopyramide

**143.** A 59-year-old male with a history of rheumatic heart disease is found to have atrial fibrillation (AF), for which he is treated with digoxin. Treatment with digoxin converts his AF to normal sinus rhythm and most likely results in a decrease in which of the following?

a. the length of the refractory period
b. the velocity of shortening of the cardiac muscle
c. conduction velocity in the atrioventricular (AV) node
d. the atrial maximum diastolic resting potential

**144.** A 65-year-old female receives digoxin and furosemide for CHF. After several months, she develops nausea and vomiting. Serum K⁺ is 2.5 mEq/L. Electrocardiogram (EKG) reveals an AV conduction defect. What cellular effect is causing these new findings?

a. increased intracellular K
b. increased intracellular guanosine 3'5'-cyclic monophosphate (cGMP)
c. increased intracellular Ca
d. increased intracellular norepinephrine
e. increased intracellular nitric oxide (NO)

$\downarrow K$     ?   $Ca$

**145.** Which of the following drugs recommended for the lowering of blood cholesterol inhibits the synthesis of cholesterol by blocking 3-hydroxy-3-methylglutaryl-coenzyme A (HMG-CoA) reductase?

a. lovastatin
b. probucol
c. clofibrate
d. gemfibrozil
e. nicotinic acid (NA)

**146.** The EKG of a patient who is receiving digitalis in the therapeutic dose range would be likely to show

a. prolongation of the QT interval
b. prolongation of the PR interval
c. symmetric peaking of the T wave
d. widening of the QRS complex
e. elevation of the ST segment

**147.** A 45-year-old male takes simvastatin for hypercholesterolemia; however, his cholesterol level remains above target at maximal doses. Cholestyramine is added to the therapeutic regimen. What drug-drug interaction can occur?

a. the combination will not lower cholesterol more than either agent alone
b. the combination causes elevated very-low-density lipoprotein (VLDL)
c. cholestyramine inhibits gastrointestinal (GI) absorption of simvastatin
d. simvastatin is a direct antagonist of cholestyramine

**148.** In a hypertensive patient who is taking insulin to treat diabetes, which of the following drugs is to be used with extra caution and advice to the patient?

a. hydralazine
b. prazosin
c. guanethidine
d. propranolol
e. methyldopa

**149.** Which of the following drugs is considered to be most effective in relieving and preventing ischemic episodes in patients with variant angina?

a. propranolol
b. nitroglycerin
c. sodium nitroprusside
d. verapamil
e. isosorbide dinitrate

**150.** A 47-year-old male is seen in the medicine clinic with recently diagnosed mixed hyperlipidemia. An antihyperlipidemic is administered that favorably affects levels of VLDL, LDL, and HDL and inhibits cholesterol synthesis. This drug is:

a. lovastatin
b. colestipol
c. niacin
d. probucol
e. neomycin

**151.** If quinidine and digoxin are administered concurrently, which of the following effects does quinidine have on digoxin?

a. the absorption of digoxin from the gastrointestinal (GI) tract is decreased
b. the metabolism of digoxin is prevented
c. the concentration of digoxin in the plasma is increased
d. the effect of digoxin on the AV node is antagonized
e. the ability of digoxin to inhibit the $Na^+,K^+$-stimulated ATPase is reduced

**152.** Drugs that block the catecholamine uptake process—such as cocaine, tricyclic antidepressants, and phenothiazines—are apt to block the antihypertensive action of which of the following drugs?

a. propranolol
b. guanethidine
c. prazosin
d. hydralazine
e. diazoxide

**153.** A 44-year-old obese male has a significantly high level of plasma triglycerides. Following treatment with one of the following agents, his plasma triglyceride levels decrease to almost normal. Which agent did he receive?

a. neomycin
b. lovastatin
c. cholestyramine
d. gemfibrozil

**154.** A 64-year-old male with arteriosclerotic heart disease (AHD) and CHF who has been treated with digoxin complains of nausea, vomiting, and diarrhea. His EKG reveals a bigeminal rhythm. The symptoms and EKG findings occurred shortly after another therapeutic agent was added to his regimen. A drug-drug interaction is suspected. Which agent was involved?

a. lovastatin
b. hydrochlorothiazide
c. phenobarbital
d. nitroglycerin
e. captopril

*(electrolyte abnormality)*

**155.** Nicotinic acid in large doses used to treat hyperlipoproteinemia causes a cutaneous flush. The vasodilatory effect is due to

a. release of histamine
b. production of local prostaglandins
c. release of platelet-derived growth factor (PDGF)
d. production of NO
e. Ca channel blockade

**156.** One type of hyperlipoproteinemia is characterized by elevated plasma levels of chylomicrons, normal plasma levels of β-lipoproteins, and the inability of any known drug to reduce lipoprotein levels. This is which of the following types of hyperlipoproteinemia?

a. type I
b. type IIa, IIb
c. type III
d. type IV
e. type V

**157.** A 69-year-old male with angina develops dizziness, headaches, lethargy, and constipation following treatment with

a. propranolol
b. captopril        *Vasodilation.*
c. nifedipine
d. dobutamine
e. nitroglycerin

**158.** ACE inhibitors are associated with a high incidence of which of the following adverse reactions?

a. hepatitis
b. hypokalemia
c. agranulocytosis
d. proteinuria
e. hirsutism

**159.** A 45-year-old male post-myocardial infarction (post-MI) for one week is being treated with intravenous (IV) heparin. Stool guaiac on admission was negative, but is now 4+, and he has had an episode of hematemesis. The heparin is discontinued, and a drug is given to counteract the bleeding. What drug was given?

*Bleeding*

a. aminocaproic acid
b. dipyridamole
c. factor IX
d. protamine
e. vitamin K

**160.** Patients with genetically low levels of N-acetyltransferase are more prone to develop a lupus erythematosus-like syndrome with which of the following drugs?

a.   propranolol
b.   procainamide
c.   digitoxin
d.   captopril
e.   lidocaine

**161.** Which of the following anemias would be treated with cyanocobalamin (vitamin $B_{12}$)?

a.   anemia in infants who are undergoing rapid growth
b.   anemia associated with cheilosis, dysphagia, gastritis, and hypochlorhydria
c.   anemia associated with small, bizarre cells poorly filled with hemoglobin (Hgb)
d.   anemia associated with infestation by D*iphyllobothrium latum*
e.   Bleeding from a gastric ulcer

**162.** The preferred agent to combat extreme digitalis overdose is

a.   K
b.   Ca
c.   phenytoin
d.   Fab fragments of digitalis antibodies
e.   magnesium (Mg)

**163.** Significant relaxation of smooth muscle of both venules and arterioles is produced by which of the following drugs?

a.   hydralazine
b.   minoxidil
c.   diazoxide
d.   sodium nitroprusside
e.   nifedipine

**164.** Precautions advisable when using lovastatin include

a.   serum transaminase measurements
b.   renal function studies
c.   acoustic measurements
d.   monthly complete blood counts
e.   avoidance of bile acid sequestrants

**165.** The first-line drug for treating an acute attack of reentrant supraventricular tachycardia (SVT) is

a.   adenosine
b.   digitalis
c.   propranolol
d.   phenylephrine
e.   edrophonium

**Questions 166–168**

For each patient, select the drug most likely to have caused the changes:

a. acetazolamide
b. amiloride
c. furosemide
d. hydrochlorothiazide
e. indapamide
f. mannitol
g. spironolactone
h. vasopressin

*b* **166.** An 83-year-old male has been effectively treated with hydrochlorothiazide to control his elevated blood pressure. He has had recent onset of weakness. Blood chemistry analysis reveals a K⁺ of 2.5 mEq/L. Another drug is added, and one month later his serum K⁺ is 4.0 mEq/L.

*↓K → ℞ amiloride*

*d* **167.** A 76-year-old male with a combined history of bronchiogenic carcinoma and CHF is maintained on a diuretic to control pulmonary and peripheral edema. Recent measurement of blood electrolytes reveals an elevated serum Ca.

*(thiazide)*

*c* **168.** A 66-year-old female with CHF and hearing loss is given a diuretic as part of a regimen that includes digoxin and an ACE inhibitor. In the course of treatment, she develops an AV conduction defect and is found to be hypomagnesemic. She also has worsening hearing loss, which is reversed when the drug is stopped.

*(furosemide)*

**DIRECTIONS:** Each numbered question or incomplete statement below is NEGATIVELY phrased. Select the **one best** lettered response.

169. Nitroglycerine, a frequently used cardiovascular drug, has all the following actions EXCEPT

a.  it can cause adverse reactions of headache and tachycardia
b.  it undergoes significant first-pass biotransformation
c.  it is used for CHF
d.  it decreases total coronary blood flow
e.  it is converted to nitrite by the smooth muscle cell

170. True statements regarding the mechanism of action of the nitrites and organic nitrates in causing smooth muscle relaxation include all the following EXCEPT

a.  NO is formed
b.  adenyl cyclase is inhibited
c.  a cyclic guanylic acid (GMP)-dependent protein kinase is stimulated
d.  the light chain of myosin is dephosphorylated
e.  the mechanism is similar to that of endothelial-derived relaxing factor (EDRF)

171. The automaticity of Purkinje's fibers of the heart can be increased by all the following EXCEPT

a.  epinephrine
b.  digitalis
c.  quinidine
d.  low K concentrations
e.  isoproterenol

172. The nitrates remain the most valuable agents for the therapy of angina pectoris. Valid statements with respect to their overall mechanism of action include all the following EXCEPT

a.  nitrates cause reflex tachycardia
b.  in normal subjects nitrates can induce a transient increase in total coronary flow by directly dilating coronary arteries
c.  in coronary artery disease beneficial actions of nitrates are attributable to a decreased myocardial oxygen requirement
d.  nitrates increase venous capacitance and thus cause a decrease in myocardial preload
e.  nitrates are incompatible with β-blockers

**173.** Endogenous heparin is characterized by all the following statements EXCEPT

a. it is found largely in mast cells
b. it is a sulfonated mucopolysaccharide
c. it is inhibited by protamine sulfate
d. it is able to release a lipemia-clearing factor
e. it crosses the placental barrier

**174.** Antiarrhythmic drugs used prophylactically to prevent sustained ventricular tachycardia may be accompanied by all the following benefits and adverse reactions EXCEPT

a. reduced number of premature ventricular contractions (PVCs)
b. elimination of runs of nonsustained ventricular tachycardia
c. torsades de pointes with class I antiarrhythmic drugs
d. prolonged life expectancy in most cases
e. relief of symptomatic premature ventricular contractions

**175.** Drugs that cause bronchodilation include all the following EXCEPT

a. theophylline
b. albuterol
c. ephedrine
d. cromolyn
e. ipratropium

**176.** A 56-year-old female has recently developed essential hypertension, for which she is receiving chlorothiazide to lower her blood pressure. Which of these ions would NOT increase in concentration in her urine?

a. $K^+$
b. $Cl^-$
c. $Ca^{++}$
d. $Na^+$
e. $Mg^{++}$

**DIRECTIONS:** Each question below contains five suggested responses. Select the **one best** response to each question.

**177.** A 60-year-old female with deep-vein thrombosis (DVT) is given a bolus of heparin, and a heparin drip is also started. Thirty minutes later, she is bleeding profusely from the IV site. The heparin is stopped, but the bleeding continues. You decide to give protamine to reverse the adverse effect of heparin. How does protamine act?

a.  it causes hydrolysis of heparin
b.  it changes the conformation of antithrombin III to prevent binding to heparin
c.  it activates the coagulation cascade, overriding the action of heparin
d.  it combines with heparin as an ion pair, inactivating it

**178.** A 47-year-old female comes to the emergency department (ED) with severe crushing chest pain of one-hour duration. EKG and blood chemistries are consistent with a diagnosis of acute MI. Streptokinase is chosen as part of the therapeutic regimen. What is its mechanism of action?

a.  it activates the conversion of fibrin to fibrin split products
b.  it activates the conversion of plasminogen to plasmin
c.  it inhibits the conversion of prothrombin to thrombin
d.  it inhibits the conversion of fibrinogen to fibrin

**Questions 179–181**

For each patient, select the drug most likely to have caused the adverse effect:

a.  adenosine
b.  captopril
c.  clonidine
d.  digoxin
e.  dobutamine
f.  furosemide
g.  guanethidine
h.  lidocaine
i.  nifedipine
j.  prazocin
k.  procainamide
l.  propranolol

**179.** A 36-year-old male is seen in the ED with tachycardia, a respiratory rate of 26 breaths per minute (BPM), and EKG evidence of an arrhythmia. An IV bolus dose of an antiarrhythmic agent is administered, and within 30 sec he has a respiratory rate of 45 BPM and complains of a burning sensation in his chest.

*diuretics*
*ideally*

*e (Dobutamine)*

**180.** Following a cardiac triple-bypass operation, a 65-year-old normotensive hospitalized female has shortness of breath, diffuse rales bilaterally, a pulse of 110/min, an elevated venous pressure, and a blood pressure of 140/85 mmHg. An IV dose of drug is given to counteract her findings. However, following administration of this drug, her pulse increases to 150/min and her blood pressure to 180/110 mmHg.

*b*

*Captopril*

**181.** A 50-year-old male with a two-year history of essential hypertension well controlled on hydrochlorothiazide is found on a recent physical examination to have a blood pressure of 160/105 mmHg. The hydrochlorothiazide is substituted with another agent. Two weeks later, he returns for follow-up complaining of loss of taste.

*a*

**182.** A 54-year-old female is treated for essential hypertension with an antihypertensive that controls her blood pressure. One day, she comes to the ED with chest pain, tachycardia, anxiety, and a blood pressure of 240/140 mmHg. She has not taken her medication for two days. Which antihypertensive can account for her findings?

a. clonidine
b. propranolol
c. doxazocin
d. minoxidil
e. prazocin

*Sympatholytic (Centrally acting)*

## Questions 183–184

For each patient, select the drug most likely to have caused the adverse effect:

a. adenosine
b. amiodarone
c. bretylium
d. flecainide
e. procainamide
f. propafenone
g. quinidine
h. sotalol
i. tocainide
j. verapamil

*Quinidine*

*g* **183.** A 68-year-old female has AF, which is treated with an antiarrhythmic agent that blocks Na channels. On a recent office visit, she complained of recurrent attacks of feeling faint and of experiencing an episode of loss of consciousness. An EKG showed marked prolongation of the QT interval. Plasma concentration of the drug was in the therapeutic range.

*Procainamide*

*e* **184.** A 55-year-old male has recurrent ventricular arrhythmias after an MI, for which he is given an antiarrhythmic agent that blocks Na channels and prolongs the action potential. One year later, a blood test is positive for circulating antinuclear antibodies.

**Questions 185–187**

Match each route of administration and treatment indication with the correct drug.

a. isoproterenol
b. terbutaline
c. nitroglycerin
d. cromolyn sodium
e. beclomethasone
f. sodium nitroprusside

*c* **185.** Administered transdermally for angina pectoris

*a* **186.** Administered parenterally to produce myocardial stimulation

*e* **187.** Administered by aerosol for bronchial asthma

**Questions 188–189**

It is customary today to classify antiarrhythmic drugs according to their mechanism of action. This is best defined by intracellular recordings that yield monophasic action potentials. In the accompanying figure, the monophasic action potentials of (A) slow response fiber (SA node) and (B) fast Purkinje fiber are shown. For each description that follows, choose the appropriate drug with which the change in character of the monophasic action potential is likely to be associated.

a. digitalis
b. amiodarone
c. mexiletine
d. nifedipine
e. propranolol
f. flecainide
g. disopyramide
h. verapamil

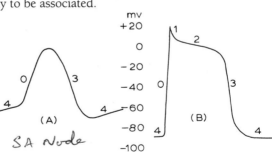

SA Node    Purkinje fibre

*g* **188.** Moderate phase 0 depression and slow conduction; prolonged repolarization

*b* **189.** Affects mainly phase 3, prolonging repolarization

( Amiodarone )

**Questions 190–192**

Match the mechanism of preventing or relieving bronchospasm with the correct drug.

a.  corticosteroids
b.  cromolyn sodium
c.  theophylline
d.  albuterol
e.  acetylcysteine
f.  ipratropium *(Atropine)*

**190.** Prevents reflex stimulation of upper and lower airways, esophagus, and carotid bodies

**191.** Breaks down sputum molecules to smaller components

**192.** Inhibits mediator release from inflammatory cells

**Questions 193–195**

Match the drugs below with the appropriate action.

a.  raises the plasma level of factor IX
b.  inhibits thrombin and early coagulation steps
c.  inhibits synthesis of prothrombin
d.  inhibits platelet aggregation in vitro
e.  activates plasminogen
f.  binds the Ca ion cofactor in some coagulation steps

**193.** Coumarin derivatives *Vit a.*

**194.** Dipyridamole *platelet a*

**195.** Ethylenediaminotetraacetic acid (EDTA) *(chelating agents)*

**Questions 196–198**

Match the descriptions below with the appropriate agent.

a.  angiotensin I
b.  angiotensin II
c.  clonidine
d.  saralasin
e.  captopril

**196.** Formed by sequential enzymatic cleavage by renin and then peptidyl dipeptidase (kinase II) *angio II*

**197.** An octapeptide that lowers blood pressure in renin-dependent hypertensive patients *(Saralasin)*

**198.** Lowers blood pressure in hypertensive patients by inhibiting peptidyl dipeptidase *(captopril)*

**199.** A 76-year-old female with an eight-year history of CHF well controlled with digoxin and furosemide develops recurrence of dyspnea on exertion. On physical examination, she has sinus tachycardia, rales at the base of both lungs, and 4+ pitting edema of the lower extremities. Which agent could be added to her therapeutic regimen?

a. dobutamine
b. hydralazine
c. minoxidil
d. prazosin
e. enalapril

**200.** A 61-year-old female has intermittent bouts of chest pain on exertion of two months' duration, associated with numbness and tingling in the fourth and fifth fingers of her left hand. EKG is normal. She is placed on propranolol, which relieves her symptoms. What cardiovascular effect did the drug have?

a. it decreased production of catecholamines
b. it dilated the coronary vasculature
c. it decreased the requirement for myocardial oxygen
d. it increased peripheral vascular resistance
e. it increased sensitivity to catecholamines

**201.** The blood pressure of a 65-year-old male is well controlled by a Ca channel-blocker used to treat his essential hypertension. When placed on cimetidine to control symptoms related to gastroesophageal reflux disease (GERD), he has episodes of dizziness. How does cimetidine's effect on Ca channel-blockers account for the dizziness?

a. it increases their rate of intestinal absorption
b. it decreases their plasma protein binding
c. it decreases their volume of distribution
d. it decreases their metabolism by cytochrome P-450
e. it decreases their tubular renal secretion

**202.** Which of the following best describes cimetidine's mechanism of interaction with procainamide?

a. it decreases procainamide metabolism
b. it decreases procainamide sensitivity at the site of action
c. it decreases procainamide renal excretion
d. it decreases procainamide plasma protein binding
e. it decreases procainamide intestinal absorption

*digoxin → Renal*
*↘ Electrolytes*

**203.** Which of the following best describes diltiazem's effect on digoxin?

a.   it decreases digoxin metabolism
b.   it decreases digoxin renal excretion
c.   it decreases digoxin plasma protein binding
d.   it decreases digoxin intestinal absorption
e.   it decreases digoxin sensitivity at its site of action

**204.** Which of the following best describes the mechanism of kaolin-pectin's interaction with digoxin?

a.   it decreases digoxin metabolism
b.   it decreases digoxin renal excretion
c.   it decreases digoxin plasma protein binding
d.   it decreases digoxin intestinal absorption
e.   it decreases digoxin sensitivity at its site of action

*201 → 204*
*Drug Interactions*   *(D) mcq*

# CARDIOVASCULAR AND PULMONARY SYSTEMS

## *Answers*

**136. The answer is d.** (*DiPalma, 4/e, pp 116–122, 133–134. Hardman and Limbird, 9/e, pp 212-213.*) Only isoproterenol will lower mean blood pressure, decrease peripheral vascular resistance, and increase heart rate. Methacholine decreases heart rate as does propranolol. Atropine has no action on peripheral resistance. Norepinephrine causes intense vasoconstriction and raises the mean blood pressure.

**137. The answer is c.** (*DiPalma, 4/e, p 390. Hardman and Limbird, 9/e, p 810.*) Digitalis inhibits Na$^+$/K$^+$ ATPase and hence decreases myocyte Na pumping, resulting in a relative reduction of Ca expulsion from Na-Ca exchange. The consequent increase in free Ca in the cell causes increased intensity of interaction between actin and myosin filaments and enhanced contractility.

**138. The answer is e.** (*DiPalma, 4/e, pp 421–423. Hardman and Limbird, 9/e, pp 858–874.*) Because verapamil, a Ca channel-blocker, has a selective depressing action on AV nodal tissue, it is an ideal drug for both immediate and prophylactic therapy of SVT. Nifedipine, another Ca channel-blocker, has little effect on supraventricular arrhythmia. Lidocaine and adenosine are parenteral drugs with short half-lives and thus are not suitable for prophylactic therapy. Procainamide is more suitable for ventricular arrhythmias and has the potential for serious adverse reactions with long-term use.

**139. The answer is c.** (*DiPalma, 4/e, pp 429–430. Hardman and Limbird, 9/e, pp 855–856.*) β-adrenergic receptor blockers cause a slowing of heart rate, lower blood pressure, and lessened cardiac contractility without reducing cardiac output. There is also a buffering action against adrenergic stimulation of the cardiac autoregulatory mechanism. These hemodynamic actions decrease the requirement of the heart for oxygen.

**140. The answer is b.** (*Hardman and Limbird, 9/e, p 697.*) The primary action of furosemide is inhibition of the $Na^+/K^+/Cl^-$ transporter in the thick ascending limb of the loop of Henle.

**141. The answer is a.** (*DiPalma, 4/e, p 472. Isselbacher, 13/e, pp 1749–1750.*) Many drugs can cause an immunohemolytic anemia. Methyldopa may cause a positive Coombs' test in as many as 20% of patients along with hemolytic anemia. Other drugs with similar actions on red blood cells are penicillins, quinidine, procainamide, and sulfonamides. These form a stable or unstable hapten on the red cell surface, which induces an immune reaction (immunoglobulin G [IgG] antibodies) and leads to dissolution of the membrane.

**142. The answer is d.** (*DiPalma, 4/e, p 415. Hardman and Limbird, 9/e, pp 865–867.*) Lidocaine usually shortens the duration of the action potential and thus allows more time for recovery during diastole. It also blocks both activated and inactivated Na channels. This has the effect of minimizing the action of lidocaine on normal myocardial tissues as contrasted to depolarized ischemic tissues. Thus lidocaine is particularly suitable for arrhythmias arising during ischemic episodes such as MI.

**143. The answer is c.** (*DiPalma, 4/e, p 394. Hardman and Limbird, 9/e, pp 813–814.*) Digoxin is used in AF to slow the ventricular rate, not usually the AF itself. Digoxin acts to slow the speed of conduction, increase the atrial and AV nodal maximal diastolic resting membrane potential, and increase the effective refractory period in the AV node, which prevents transmission of all impulses from the atria to the ventricles. It exerts these effects by directly acting on the heart and by indirectly increasing vagal activity.

**144. The answer is c.** (*Katzung, 7/e, pp 203–204.*) Overloading of cell Ca leads to "delayed afterdepolarizations." These afterpotentials can interfere with normal conduction by further reducing the resting potential; if they regularly reach threshold in the conduction system, an arrhythmia can occur.

**145. The answer is a.** (*DiPalma, 4/e, p 450. Hardman and Limbird, 9/e, pp 885–887.*) Lovastatin decreases cholesterol synthesis in the liver by inhibiting HMG-CoA reductase, the rate-limiting enzyme in the synthetic pathway. This results in an increase in LDL receptors in the liver, thus reducing blood levels for cholesterol. The intake of dietary cholesterol must not be increased, as this would allow the liver to use more exogenous cholesterol and defeat the action of lovastatin.

**146. The answer is b.** (DiPalma, 4/e, p 391. Hardman and Limbird, 9/e, pp 813–814.) The usual electrocardiographic pattern of a patient receiving therapeutic doses of digitalis includes an increase in the PR interval, depression and sagging of the ST segment, and occasional biphasia or inversion of the T wave. Symmetrically peaked T waves are associated with hyperkalemia or ischemia in most cases. Shortening of the QT interval, rather than prolongation, is characteristic of digitalis treatment.

**147. The answer is c.** (Hardman and Limbird, 9/e, pp 887, 889.) Bile acid-binding resins bind more than just bile acids, and binding of simvastatin to cholestyramine is the most likely mechanism for decreased GI absorption. Cholestyramine may also bind to several other drugs, including digitalis, benzothiadiazides (thiazides), warfarin, vancomycin, thyroxine ($T_4$), and aspirin. Medications should be given one hour before or four hours after cholestyramine.

**148. The answer is d.** (DiPalma, 4/e, p 136. Hardman and Limbird, 9/e, pp 855–856.) Propranolol as well as other nonselective β-blockers tends to slow the rate of recovery in a hypoglycemic attack caused by insulin. β-blockers also mask the symptoms of hypoglycemia and may actually cause hypertension because of the increased plasma epinephrine in the presence of vascular $\beta_2$ blockade.

**149. The answer is d.** (DiPalma, 4/e, pp 434–435. Hardman and Limbird, 9/e, pp 767–775.) Ca channel-blockers, of which nifedipine is a prime example, are now considered to be more effective than nitrates in relieving variant angina. This is because this type of angina is believed to be caused by vasospasm, which is best antagonized by slow channel Ca blockers. Such blockers appear to have a relative selectivity for coronary arteries.

**150. The answer is c.** (Hardman and Limbird, 9/e, p 890. Katzung, 7/e, p 570.) Only niacin improves levels of VLDL, HDL, and LDL and inhibits the cholesterol synthesis. It also limits the progression of atherosclerosis by lowering circulating fibrinogen and increasing circulating tPA.

**151. The answer is c.** *(DiPalma, 4/e, p 395. Hardman and Limbird, 9/e, pp 870–871.)* Quinidine is often given in conjunction with digitalis. It has been found by pharmacokinetic studies that this combination results in quinidine's replacing digitalis in tissue binding sites (mainly muscle), thus raising the blood level of digitalis and decreasing its volume of distribution. A mechanism by which quinidine interferes with the renal excretion of digitalis has also been proposed.

**152. The answer is b.** *(DiPalma, 4/e, p 144. Hardman and Limbird, 9/e, p 790.)* Neuronal uptake is necessary for the hypotensive action of guanethidine. It competes for the norepinephrine storage site and in time replaces the natural neurotransmitter. This is the basis of its hypotensive effect. Drugs that prevent reuptake by the neurons, such as cocaine, would destroy the effectiveness of guanethidine.

**153. The answer is d.** *(Katzung, 7/e, pp 571–572.)* Only gemfibrozil acts to lower triglycerides, probably because of increased lipolysis by lipoprotein lipase and decreased lipolysis inside adipocytes, causing a net movement of triglycerides into the cell.

**154. The answer is b.** *(DiPalma, 4/e, p 356. Hardman and Limbird, 9/e, pp 703–704.)* Low K stores due to the effects of thiazide diuretics such as hydrochlorothiazide increase susceptibility to cardiac glycoside toxicity.

**155. The answer is b.** *(DiPalma, 4/e, p 447. Hardman and Limbird, 9/e, pp 890–891.)* Nicotinic acid (NA) in large doses stimulates the production of prostaglandins as shown by an increase in blood level. The flush may be prevented by the prior administration of aspirin, which is known to block synthesis of prostaglandins.

**156. The answer is a.** *(DiPalma, 4/e, pp 444–445. Hardman and Limbird, 9/e, pp 875–898.)* In type I hyperlipoproteinemia, drugs that reduce levels of lipoproteins are not useful, but reduction of dietary sources of fat may help. Cholesterol levels are usually normal but triglycerides are elevated. Maintenance of ideal body weight is recommended in all types of hyperlipidemia. Clofibrate effectively reduces the levels of very low-density lipoproteins characteristic of types III, IV, and V hyperlipoproteinemias; and administration of cholestyramine resin and lovastatin in conjunction with a low-cholesterol diet is regarded as effective therapy for type IIa, or primary, hyperbeta-lipoproteinemia, except in the homozygous familial form.

**157. The answer is c.** (*Hardman and Limbird, 9/e, p 772.*) Excessive vasodilation is a common adverse effect of Ca channel-blockers such as nifedipine This can cause dizziness, hypotension, headache, flushing, nausea, and diminished sensation in fingers and toes. Constipation, lethargy, nervousness, and peripheral edema are also seen with the use of these drugs.

**158. The answer is d.** (*DiPalma, 4/e, p 481. Hardman and Limbird, 9/e, p 750.*) The most consistent of the toxicities of inhibitors of ACEs is impairment of renal function evidenced by proteinuria. Elevations of blood urea nitrogen (BUN), and creatinine occur frequently, especially when stenosis of the renal artery or severe heart failure exists. Hyperkalemia also may occur. These drugs are to be used very cautiously where prior renal failure is present and in the elderly. Other toxicities include neutropenia and angioedema. Hepatic toxicity has not been reported.

**159. The answer is d.** (*Hardman and Limbird, 9/e, p 1346.*) A slow IV infusion of protamine sulfate will quickly reverse the bleeding. Protamine binds to heparin to form a stable complex with no anticoagulant activity. It may also have its own anticoagulant effect by binding with platelets and fibrinogen.

**160. The answer is b.** (*DiPalma, 4/e, pp 413–414. Hardman and Limbird, 9/e, pp 868–869.*) Persons with low hepatic N-acetyltransferase activity are known as slow acetylators. A major pathway of metabolism of procainamide, which is used to treat arrhythmias, is N-acetylation. Slow acetylators receiving this drug are more susceptible than normal persons to side effects, since slow acetylators will have higher-than-normal blood levels of these drugs. N-Acetylprocainamide, the metabolite of procainamide, is also active.

**161. The answer is d.** (*DiPalma, 4/e, pp 507, 516. Hardman and Limbird, 9/e, pp 1331–1333.*) Fe deficiency anemia usually occurs in infants undergoing rapid growth. In adults in a late stage it may result in a bowel syndrome associated with gastritis and hypochlorhydria (Plummer-Vinson syndrome). Characteristically all Fe deficiency anemias are associated with a hypochromic microcytic blood profile. Infestation with the tapeworm *D. latum* is accompanied by a hyperchromic macrocytic anemia treatable with vitamin $B_{12}$. Bleeding syndromes are treated with Fe.

**162. The answer is d.** (_DiPalma, 4/e, p 396. Hardman and Limbird, 9/e, p 820._) In digitalis overdose only the administration of a specific Fab fragment that acts as an antibody for digitalis is effective. This raises the blood level of the digitalis glycoside but it is not available for action on the heart and indeed the combined Fab fragment–digitalis complex is excreted by the kidney. While K, Mg, and phenytoin will counteract some of the arrhythmogenic actions of digitalis, they are not effective in severe digitalis overdose. Ca would augment the toxicity of digitalis.

**163. The answer is d.** (_DiPalma, 4/e, pp 397–398. Hardman and Limbird, 9/e, pp 794–795._) Hydralazine, minoxidil, diazoxide, and sodium nitroprusside are all directly acting vasodilators used to treat hypertension. Because hydralazine, minoxidil, nifedipine, and diazoxide relax arteriolar smooth muscle more than smooth muscle in venules, the effect on venous capacitance is negligible. Sodium nitroprusside, which affects both arterioles and venules, does not increase cardiac output, a feature that enhances the utility of sodium nitroprusside in the management of hypertensive crisis associated with MI.

**164. The answer is a.** (_DiPalma, 4/e, pp 450–452. Hardman and Limbird, 9/e, pp 885–887._) Lovastatin should not be used in patients with severe liver disease. With routine use of lovastatin, serum transaminase values may rise, and in such patients the drug may be continued only with great caution. Lovastatin has also been associated with lenticular opacities, and slit-lamp studies should be done before and 1 year after the start of therapy. There is no effect on the otic nerve. The drug is not toxic to the renal system and reports of bone marrow depression are very rare. There is a small incidence of myopathy, and levels of creatinine kinase should be measured when unexplained muscle pain occurs. Combination with cyclosporine or clofibrate has led to myopathy. There is no danger in use with bile acid sequestrants.

**165. The answer is a.** (_DiPalma, 4/e, pp 421–423. Isselbacher, 13/e, pp 1026–1027, 1032._) Older therapies—all designed to favor parasympathetic control of rhythm—include digitalis, propranolol, edrophonium, and vasoconstrictors. The vasoconstrictor phenylephrine (given by intravenous bolus) causes stimulation of the carotid sinus and reflex vagal stimulation of the atria. More recently, adenosine has been favored over verapamil, which is also very effective but slower acting.

**166. The answer is b.** (_DiPalma, 4/e, pp 463–465._) Amiloride is a K-sparing diuretic with a mild diuretic and natriuretic effect. The parent compound is active, and the drug is excreted unchanged in the urine. Amiloride has a 24-hour duration of action and is usually administered with a thiazide or loop diuretic (e.g., furosemide) to prevent hypokalemia. The site of its diuretic action is the late distal tubule and collecting duct, where it interferes with Na reabsorption and allows for K retention.

**167. The answer is d.** *(Katzung, 7/e, p 251.)* Thiazide diuretics raise serum Ca, possibly through a direct effect on Ca reabsorption in the distal tubule and reabsorption in the proximal tubule from volume depletion. While rarely caused by the diuretic alone, hypercalcemia can occur when the patient has a history of carcinoma.

**168. The answer is c.** *(Katzung, 7/e, pp 249–251.)* Furosemide can cause hypokalemia by blocking Na⁺ reabsorption in the loop of Henle, followed by exchange of K⁺ with Na⁺ in the distal tubules. Hypokalemia is associated with digitalis toxicity. Furosemide also can cause dose-related hearing loss, especially in people with existing hearing loss and/or renal impairment.

**169. The answer is d.** *(DiPalma, 4/e, pp 425–428. Hardman and Limbird, 9/e, pp 761–765.)* Nitroglycerine is the most frequently administered antianginal drug. Its main adverse effects are headache and tachycardia in many patients. By the oral route it undergoes very active first-pass biotransformation and thus is very short-acting. Recently, it has been frequently employed in CHF because of its property of dilating the venous bed. Despite the fact that nitrates do dilate coronary vessels, most studies show that total coronary flow is not increased (it certainly is not decreased). The sulfhydryl (SH) group in myocyte membranes converts nitrate to nitrite.

**170. The answer is b.** *(DiPalma, 4/e, pp 427–428. Hardman and Limbird, 9/e, p 764.)* Adenyl cyclase is not involved. The receptor for nitrite converts NO₂ to NO. This free radical reacts with guanylate cyclase to cause increased synthesis of guanosine 3′,-5′ cyclic monophosphate (cyclic cGMP). A GMP-dependent protein kinase is activated; this results in decreased phosphorylation of muscle protein, which decreases the muscle's capacity to contract. In this manner, nitrates relax all smooth muscles. This action of nitrites is identical to that of EDRF.

**171. The answer is c.** *(DiPalma, 4/e, pp 119, 405, 410. Hardman and Limbird, 9/e, pp 869–870.)* Automaticity of Purkinje's fibers is increased by epinephrine, digitalis, isoproterenol, and low concentration of K. It is decreased by quinidine or high concentration of K. The modification of automaticity is important: in complete heart block, a condition of rhythm failure with bradycardia, isoproterenol or epinephrine might be used to enhance the automaticity of the ventricular conductive system. However, in the situation of supraventricular and ventricular ectopy, all agents able to facilitate automaticity should be avoided.

**172. The answer is e.** (*DiPalma, 4/e, pp 425–427. Hardman and Limbird, 9/e, pp 761–765.*) There is no doubt that, experimentally, nitrates dilate coronary vessels. This also occurs in normal subjects, resulting in an overall increase in coronary blood flow. In arteriosclerotic coronaries, the ability to dilate is lost and the ischemic area may actually have less blood flow under the influence of nitrates. Improvement in the ischemic condition is the result of decreased myocardial oxygen demands because of a reduction of preload and afterload. Nitrates dilate both arteries and veins, and thus reduce the work of the heart. As the blood pressure falls, there is reflex tachycardia. Nitrates are compatible with β-blockers, which slow the heart and counteract the reflex tachycardia caused by nitrates.

**173. The answer is e.** (*DiPalma, 4/e, pp 526–528. Hardman and Limbird, 9/e, pp 1343–1345.*) Heparin, a naturally occurring anticoagulant, is localized largely in mast cells. A mucopolysaccharide, it is composed of sulfated glucosamine and glucuronic acid. Its primary action is as an antithrombin factor, for which it requires a plasma cofactor. Organic bases (protamine) are believed to inhibit heparin by neutralizing its electronegative charge. Heparin is thought to release and stabilize a lipemia-clearing factor that catalyzes the hydrolysis of triglycerides. It does not cross the placental barrier and thus can be used as an anticoagulant during pregnancy.

**174. The answer is d.** (*DiPalma, 4/e, pp 422–423. Isselbacher, 13/e, pp 1031–1034.*) Although antiarrhythmic drugs are capable of reducing the number of premature ventricular contractions and even eliminating nonsustained ventricular tachycardia, they do not prolong life. This was conclusively shown in the Cardiac Arrhythmia Suppression Trial (CAST), a large-scale study that compared use of antiarrhythmic agents against placebo. Class I antiarrhythmic drugs are apt to cause proarrhythmic changes as well as torsades de pointes. Longevity in cardiac disease is related more closely to the degree of depression of the ejection fraction than to the incidence of arrhythmias.

**175. The answer is d.** (*DiPalma, 4/e, pp 489–490. Hardman and Limbird, 9/e, p 668.*) Cromolyn does not relax bronchial or other smooth muscle. In fact it may on rare occasions cause bronchospasm. It is used prophylactically rather than acutely in an asthmatic attack. Cromolyn does reduce bronchial hyper-responsiveness, presumably by inhibiting antigen-induced bronchospasm. The exact role played by its ability to stabilize mast cells is not clear.

**176. The answer is c.** (*DiPalma, 4/e, pp 457–458. Katzung, 7/e, p 251.*) Thiazide diuretics enhance K, Cl, Na, and Mg ion excretion; Ca excretion appears to be reduced following chronic drug administration. Because thiazides inhibit NaCl reabsorption in the early portion of the distal tubule, an increased load of Na and Cl ions is presented to the collecting duct, where some Na ions may be actively reabsorbed and K ions secreted, leading to increased K loss.

**177. The answer is d.** (*Hardman and Limbird, 9/e, p 1346.*) Heparin is a mixture of sulfated mucopolysaccharides and is highly acidic and highly charged. Protamine is a very basic polypeptide that combines with heparin, and the complex has no anticoagulant activity. Excess protamine does have anticoagulant activity, so just enough should be given to counteract the heparin effect.

**178. The answer is b.** (*Hardman and Limbird, 9/e, p 1352.*) Streptokinase forms a stable complex with plasminogen. The resulting conformational change allows for formation of free plasmin, the active fibrinolytic enzyme.

**179. The answer is a.** (*Hardman and Limbird, 9/e, p 858. Katzung, 7/e, p 237.*) Many patients that receive a therapeutic dose of adenosine experience shortness of breath and fullness or a burning sensation in the chest. These adverse effects are of short duration because of rapid elimination of the drug.

**180. The answer is e.** (*Hardman and Limbird, 9/e, p 213.*) IV infusion of dobutamine may result in an increased heart rate and blood pressure. Patients with a history of hypertension are more likely to have an exaggerated blood pressure response. Thorough H/o IM palpats

**181. The answer is b.** (*Hardman and Limbird, 9/e, pp 750–751.*) ACE inhibitors, especially captopril, can cause alteration or loss of taste sensation.

**182. The answer is a.** (*Hardman and Limbird, 9/e, p 789. Katzung, 7/e, pp 160–161.*) Withdrawal of clonidine, particularly doses greater than 1 mg/day, is well known to cause such a syndrome (including severe hypertension, tachycardia, anxiety, tremor, headache, abdominal pain, and sweating), even after one or two missed doses.

**183. The answer is g.** *(Hardman and Limbird, 9/e, p 870. Katzung, 7/e, p 227.)* Quinidine causes prolongation of the QT interval at therapeutic doses, possibly because of its antimuscarinic actions. In some patients, this is associated with recurrent lightheadedness and fainting ("quinidine syncope").

**184. The answer is e.** *(Hardman and Limbird, 9/e, p 868. Katzung, 7/e, pp 228–230.)* Procainamide blocks open $Na^+$ channels. Long-term therapy can result in drug-induced lupus syndrome identified by circulating antinuclear antibodies. Many patients may develop a facial rash and joint pains. Pericarditis can occur, but renal involvement is rare.

**185–187. The answers are 185-c, 186-a, 187-e.** *(DiPalma, 4/e, pp 118, 122, 398, 490. Hardman and Limbird, 9/e, pp 212, 214, 666, 764, 800.)* Isoproterenol, a catecholamine that acts on β-adrenergic receptors, is given parenterally because absorption after sublingual or oral administration is unreliable. It is a synthetic sympathomimetic structurally similar to epinephrine. Isoproterenol produces myocardial stimulation and is used for the treatment of AV heart block, cardiogenic shock associated with MI, cardiac arrest, and septicemic shock.

Terbutaline is a synthetic sympathomimetic amine that acts on the β-adrenergic receptors of bronchial smooth muscle and causes a decrease in airway and pulmonary resistance. Oral doses are effective for management of bronchial asthma and for the reversible bronchospasm that may occur in bronchitis and emphysema. Terbutaline has a modest therapeutic advantage over a less selective bronchodilator.

The coronary vasodilator nitroglycerine may be administered orally, sublingually, topically, intravenously, and most recently transdermally. Its small dose and molecular structure permit its passage through the skin. This is accomplished by attaching a nitroglycerine-containing, multilayered film to the skin.

Beclomethasone is a glucocorticoid especially designed for aerosol administration. This permits its therapeutic action in the lungs while minimizing systemic effects. Great care must be exercised when transferring patients from systemic corticosteroids to beclomethasone because fatal adrenal insufficiency has occurred in asthmatic patients undergoing such transfer.

Sodium nitroprusside can only be administered intravenously. It is an effective vasodilator for heart failure because it dilates both arterioles and veins and thus reduces both preload and afterload. Maximal onset of action is in 1 to 2 min, and the effect dissipates rapidly when infusion is stopped.

Cromolyn sodium is inhaled as a powder administered by a special device ("turbo-inhaler").

**188–189. The answers are 188-g, 189-b.** (*DiPalma, 4/e, pp 401, 410. Hardman and Limbird, 9/e, pp 858–859, 864–865.*) It is widely accepted that antiarrhythmic drugs are best classified according to their electrophysiologic attributes. This is best accomplished by relating the effects of the different drugs to their actions on Na and Ca channels, which are reflected by changes in the monophasic action potential. Amiodarone blocks Na channels and markedly prolongs repolarization, particularly in depolarized cells. Flecainide is related to local anesthetics and also affects Na channels, but has little effect on repolarization. Mexiletine, which is in the same group of local anesthetics as lidocaine, is remarkable because it either does not affect or shortens repolarization. Its action is mainly on depolarized fibers. Disopyramide slows depolarization and repolarization and, like quinidine, delays conduction. Verapamil, a Ca channel-blocker, affects the resting potential or phase 4 and thus has its greatest effect on pacemaker tissue; it is mainly of utility in supraventricular arrhythmias. Digitalis also affects phase 4 of the action potential, but it also greatly hastens repolarization. Although nifedipine is a Ca channel-blocker, it has little effect on the electrophysiology of the heart. Propranolol has actions mainly on slow-response fibers and suppresses automaticity.

**190–192. The answers are 190-f, 191-e, 192-b.** (*DiPalma, 4/e, pp 486–498. Hardman and Limbird, 9/e, pp 154–155, 667–668.*) Acetylcholine is the motor for the smooth muscle of the bronchi, and ipratropium appears to inhibit vagally mediated reflexes by antagonizing the action of acetylcholine. Reflex α stimuli carried over the vagus nerve cause bronchospasm. Actually ipratropium is of little use in asthma but is effective in COPD. Acetylcysteine, known as a mucolytic, breaks the fibrillar molecules of mucoproteins by breaking down disulfide bridges of glycoproteins. It is useful in dissolution and expectoration of bronchial inflammatory products.

Cromolyn, a mast cell stabilizer, also inhibits the release of inflammatory agents (leukotrienes) from other inflammatory cells. It has anti-platelet-activating activity as well.

**193–195. The answers are 193-c, 194-d, 195-f.** (*DiPalma, 4/e, pp 437, 528–530, 533–534, 831–832. Hardman and Limbird, 9/e, pp 1347–1348, 1353–1354, 1664–1665.*) Coumarin derivatives antagonize vitamin K and cause a decrease in production of prothrombin and coagulation factors VII, IX, and X. Oral anticoagulants prevent formation of these factors by blocking formation of the reduced form of vitamin K.

Dipyridamole is classified as a coronary vasodilator. Its effectiveness in inhibiting platelet aggregation and adhesion has been proved in vitro but has still to be demonstrated in vivo. Dipyridamole is used in patients with prosthetic heart valves as primary prophylaxis against thromboemboli. It is used in combination with warfarin.

EDTA inactivates Ca in vitro by forming a complex with the Ca, thus preventing clotting. This approach is impossible in vivo because Ca levels that are low enough to prevent coagulation also are low enough to be lethal.

**196–198. The answers are 196-b, 197-d, 198-e.** *(DiPalma, 4/e, pp 470, 479–482. Hardman and Limbird, 9/e, pp 736, 741,743–745.)* The enzyme renin acts upon angiotensinogen (an α-globulin) to yield the decapeptide angiotensin I, which has limited pharmacologic activity. Angiotensin I is metabolized extensively in a single passage through the lungs by the carboxypeptidase peptidyl dipeptidase (kinase II, or ACE) to the octapeptide angiotensin II.

Angiotensin II has a potent direct action on the vascular smooth muscle and also indirectly stimulates contraction by means of the sympathetic nervous system. The vasoconstriction in response to angiotensin II involves precapillary arterioles and postcapillary venules and results in an increased total peripheral resistance.

The octapeptide saralasin is an analogue of angiotensin II and has an alanine in place of the phenylalanine in the 8 position. It is a potent antagonist of angiotensin II and, thus, can reduce elevated blood pressure in patients with significant amounts of circulating angiotensin II (i.e., renin-dependent hypertension). Being a polypeptide, saralasin must be administered intravenously, which limits its therapeutic use.

Captopril and clonidine, in contrast, are orally effective antihypertensive agents. Captopril (1-[(25)-3-mercapto-2-methylpropinoyl]-L-proline) is a rationally designed, competitive inhibitor of peptidyl dipeptidase. Unlike saralasin, it blocks the formation but not the response of angiotensin II. Captopril is useful in reducing the blood pressure of both renin-dependent and normal-renin essential hypertension. The hypotensive action of clonidine is believed to be due primarily to stimulation of the α-adrenergic receptors in the central nervous system (CNS). A reduction in the discharge rate of preganglionic adrenergic nerves occurs in addition to bradycardia.

The CNS actions of clonidine also lead to a reduction in the level of renin activity in the plasma.

**199. The answer is e.** (*DiPalma, 4/e, pp 397–398. Hardman and Limbird, 9/e, p 745.*) Vasodilator therapy for CHF has gained prominence in the past 10 years. The ACE inhibitors, such as enalapril, are among the best agents for this purpose, although Ca channel inhibitors and nitroglycerin can also be used. The ACE inhibitors dilate arterioles and veins (reducing preload), as well as inhibit aldosterone production (reducing blood volume), factors considered beneficial in CHF therapy.

**200. The answer is c.** (*DiPalma, 4/e, pp 429–430. Hardman and Limbird, 9/e, pp 774–775.*) β-adrenergic receptor-blockers slow heart rate, lower blood pressure, and lessen cardiac contractility without reducing cardiac output; they also have a buffering action against adrenergic stimulation of the cardiac autoregulatory mechanism. These hemodynamic actions decrease the requirement of the heart for oxygen.

**201. The answer is d.** (*Hardman and Limbird, 9/e, p 906.*) Cimetidine slows the metabolism of Ca channel-blockers, which are substrates for hepatic mixed-function oxidases. Inhibition of cytochrome P-450 activity is peculiar to cimetidine, and is not a mechanism of action of other histamine$_2$ (H$_2$) blockers.

**202. The answer is c.** (*Hardman and Limbird, 9/e, p 906. Katzung, 7/e, pp 1064–1065.*) Cimetidine inhibits proximal tubular secretion of procainamide, resulting in increased plasma concentrations of procainamide and its active metabolite, N-acetylprocainamide.

**203. The answer is b.** (*Hardman and Limbird, 9/e, pp 816–818.*) Digoxin levels rise with concomitant administration of diltiazem by an unknown mechanism that reduces renal clearance.

**204. The answer is d.** (*Hardman and Limbird, 9/e, pp 816–818.*) Digoxin levels can be reduced by 25% with concomitant use of kaolin-pectin by an unknown mechanism that decreases GI absorption.

# CENTRAL NERVOUS SYSTEM

**Note: In the classification of drugs, prototype drugs are marked with an asterisk (*).**

General Anesthetics
  Halothane*
  Euflurane*
  Isoflurane
  Methoxyflurane
  Nitrous oxide ($N_2O$)
  Desflurane
  Sevoflurane
Intravenous (IV) Anesthetics
  Thiopental*
  Methohexital
  Midazolam
  Ketamine
  Etomidate
  Fentanyl
  Propofol
Sedatives and Hypnotics
  Barbiturates
    Amobarbital
    Butabarbital
    Secobarbital
    Mephobarbital
    Metharbital
    Phenobarbital*
  Benzodiazepines
    Flurazepam*
    Temazepam
    Triazolam
    Quazepam

Estazolam
Miscellaneous group
  Chloral hydrate
  Paraldehyde
  Ethchlorvynol
  Ethinamate
  Glutethimide
  Zolpidem
Antianxiety Drugs
  Benzodiazepines
    Chlordiazepoxide*
    Diazepam*
    Clorazepate
    Halazepam
    Lorazepam
    Oxazepam
    Prazepam
    Alprazolam
  Propanediols
    Meprobamate*
  Miscellaneous
    Buspirone
    Hydroxyzine
Ethanol and Related Alcohols
  Ethanol*
  Ethylene glycol
  Isopropyl alcohol
  Methanol
  Disulfiram as a deterrent

Psychotomimetic Drugs
  Lysergic acid diethylamide (LSD)*
  Mescaline
  Psilocybin
  Phencyclidine
  Amphetamine
  Methamphetamine
  Cocaine*
  Marijuana*
Antipsychotic Drugs
  Phenothiazines
    Promazine
    Chlorpromazine*
    Triflupromazine
    Prochlorperazine
    Trifluoperazine
    Fluphenazine
    Thioridazine
  Thioxanthene derivatives
    Chlorprothixene
    Thiothixene
  Butyrophenone
    Haloperidol*
  Miscellaneous group
    Molindone
    Loxapine
    Pimozide
    Lithium carbonate
Antidepressant Drugs
  Tricyclics
    Imipramine*
    Amitriptyline
    Desipramine
    Nortriptyline
    Protriptyline
    Trimipramine
    Doxepin
  Monoamine oxidase inhibitors
    Tranylcypromine*

  Phenelzine
  Isocarboxazid
Second-generation antidepressants
  Maprotiline
  Amoxapine
  Trazodone
  Fluoxetine*
  Sertraline
  Paroxetine
Antiepileptic and Antiparkinsonism
  Drugs
  Tonic-clonic and focal seizures
    Phenytoin,* mephenytoin
    Carbamazepine
    Phenobarbital
    Primidone
  Absence seizures
    Ethosuximide*
    Valproic acid*
    Clonazepam
    Trimethadione
    Gabapentin
  Anticholinergics for parkinsonism
    Trihexyphenidyl*
    Procyclidine
    Biperiden
    Benztropine*
    Diphenhydramine
    Orphenadrine
  Levodopa (L-dopa) for parkin-
    sonism
    Selegiline*
  Miscellaneous agents for parkin-
    sonism
    Amantadine
    Bromocriptine*
Narcotic Analgesics
  Endogenous opioid peptides
    Met- and leu-enkephalin

β-Endorphin
Dynorphin
Agonists
  Morphine*
  Codeine*
  Heroin
  Hydromorphone
  Oxymorphone
  Oxycodone
  Levorphanol
  Meperidine, methadone
  Propoxyphene
Antagonists
  Naloxone*
  Naltrexone*
  Mixed agonists-antagonists
    Buprenorphine
    Butorphanol
    Nalbuphine
    Pentazocine
    Dezocine
Local Anesthetics
  Esters
    Cocaine*

Procaine*
Chloroprocaine
Tetracaine
Amides
  Lidocaine*
  Mepivacaine
  Bupivacaine
  Etidocaine
  Prilocaine
Drug Dependence
  Terms
    Psychological dependence
    Addiction
    Physical dependence
    Drug abuse
    Tolerance
Schedules of Drug Enforcement
    Administration
  Numbers I to VI
Stimulants
  Cocaine and amphetamines
  Hallucinogens (e.g., LSD)
  Marijuana

# Questions

**DIRECTIONS:** Each question below contains several suggested responses. Select the **one best** response to each question.

**205.** An ex-heroin addict is maintained on methadone, but succumbs to temptation and buys an opioid on the street. He takes it and rapidly goes into withdrawal. Which opioid did he take?

a. meperidine
b. heroin
c. pentazocine
d. codeine
e. propoxyphene

**206.** Which of the following opioid agonists is only administered by the parenteral route?

a. morphine
b. codeine
c. fentanyl
d. methadone
e. propoxyphene

**207.** Which of the following local anesthetics is useful for topical (surface) administration only?

a. procaine
b. bupivacaine
c. etidocaine
d. benzocaine
e. lidocaine

**208.** Akathisia, Parkinson-like syndrome, galactorrhea, and amenorrhea are side effects of perphenazine caused by

a. blockade of muscarinic receptors
b. blockade of α-adrenergic receptors
c. blockade of dopamine receptors
d. supersensitivity of dopamine receptors
e. stimulation of nicotinic receptors

**209.** Which of the following agents is useful in treatment of malignant hyperthermia?

a. baclofen
b. diazepam
c. cyclobenzaprine
d. dantrolene
e. halothane

**210.** Inhibitors of serotonin (5-HT) uptake like paroxetine interact significantly with which of the following drugs?

a. chlorpromazine
b. tranylcypromine
c. halothane
d. benztropine
e. digitalis

**211.** Which of the following is an antidepressant agent that selectively inhibits serotonin (5-HT) uptake with minimal effect on norepinephrine uptake?

a.  protriptyline
b.  maprotiline
c.  fluoxetine
d.  desipramine
e.  amoxapine

**212.** Which of the following inhalation anesthetics is most likely to produce hepatotoxicity?

a.  isoflurane
b.  enflurane
c.  methoxyflurane
d.  halothane
e.  nitrous oxide

**213.** Carbidopa is useful in the treatment of Parkinson's disease because it

a.  is a precursor of levodopa
b.  is a dopaminergic receptor agonist
c.  prevents peripheral biotransformation of L-dopa
d.  prevents breakdown of dopamine
e.  promotes a decreased concentration of L-dopa in the nigrostriatum

**214.** Which of the following is described as a competitive benzodiazepine receptor antagonist?

a.  ketamine
b.  chlordiazepoxide
c.  flumazenil
d.  midazolam
e.  triazolam

**215.** Which of the following drugs mimics the activity of metenkephalin in the dorsal horn of the spinal cord?

a.  deprenyl (selegiline)
b.  trihexyphenidyl
c.  baclofen
d.  morphine
e.  phenobarbital

**216.** The preferred treatment of status epilepticus is IV administration of

a.  chlorpromazine
b.  diazepam
c.  succinylcholine
d.  tranylcypromine
e.  ethosuximide

**217.** The most common adverse effect associated with the tricyclic antidepressants is

a.  anticholinergic effects
b.  seizures
c.  arrhythmias
d.  hepatotoxicity
e.  nephrotoxicity

**218.** A 25-year-old male is seen in the emergency department (ED). He is disoriented, but states that he has had nausea, vomiting, abdominal pain, and diarrhea since he took "too many pain pills." Before he can tell you more, he loses consciousness. Liver function tests are abnormal. In addition to gastric lavage, what is the appropriate treatment?

a.  naloxone
b.  diphenoxylate
c.  N-acetylcysteine
d.  prochlorperazine
e.  pralidoxime

**219.** Which of the following is a selective inhibitor of monoamine oxidase type B (MAO-B) and is therefore useful in treating parkinsonism?

a.   bromocriptine
b.   carbidopa
c.   selegiline
d.   phenelzine
e.   tranylcypromine

**220.** Which of the following statements is true concerning abuse of opioid analgesics?

a.   no cross tolerance develops among opioid analgesics
b.   tolerance develops equally to all effects of opioids
c.   opioids reduce pain, aggression, and sexual drives
d.   the symptoms of acute methadone withdrawal are qualitatively different from those of acute heroin withdrawal
e.   none of the above

**221.** A 36-year-old male heroin addict is seen in the ED because he cannot be aroused from sleep. On examination, he has shallow breathing and pinpoint pupils. Naloxone is administered, and the patient wakes up. Which of the opiate receptor subtypes that binds naloxone is responsible for reversing the respiratory depression and miosis?

a.   δ
b.   κ
c.   μ

**222.** A drug that specifically enhances metabolically the activity of brain dopamine is

a.   benztropine
b.   selegiline
c.   trihexyphenidyl
d.   bromocriptine
e.   chlorpromazine

**223.** A dopamine receptor agonist useful in the therapy of Parkinson's disease is

a.   selegiline
b.   bromocriptine
c.   apomorphine
d.   amantidine
e.   belladonna

**224.** In addition to its use in the treatment of schizophrenia, chlorpromazine is effective

a.   in reducing nausea and vomiting
b.   as an antihypertensive agent
c.   as an antihistaminic
d.   in the treatment of depression
e.   for treating bipolar affective disorder

**225.** Morphine may be best characterized by which of the following statements?

a.   it is classified as a mixed agonist-antagonist drug
b.   it inhibits withdrawal symptoms in persons dependent on heroin
c.   at high doses it causes death by respiratory depression
d.   it is a pure opioid antagonist at the μ, κ, and δ receptors
e.   it has an addiction potential equal to that of codeine

**226.** Cocaine, produced from the leaves of *Erythroxylon* species,

a. produces bradycardia and vasodilation
b. is directly related chemically to opioid analgesics
c. is metabolized by the microsomal metabolizing system
d. effectively blocks nerve conduction
e. blocks norepinephrine receptors directly

**227.** Which of the following agents is a selective dopamine receptor ($D_2$) agonist? *(repeat a)*

a. fluphenazine
b. bromocriptine
c. promethazine
d. haloperidol
e. chlorpromazine

**228.** Haloperidol may best be characterized by which of the following statements?

a. it is classified as a phenothiazine
b. it is a selective $D_2$ receptor agonist
c. its mechanism of action is completely different from that of chlorpromazine
d. it is more potent as an antipsychotic drug than is chlorpromazine
e. it produces a lower incidence of extrapyramidal reactions than does chlorpromazine

**229.** A 33-year-old female patient treated with haloperidol for a history of schizophrenia is seen in the ED because of complaints of fever, stiffness, and tremor. Her temperature is 104°F, and her serum creatine kinase (CK) level is elevated. What has occurred? (b)

a. overdose
b. allergy
c. neuroleptic malignant syndrome (NMS)
d. tardive dyskinesia
e. parkinsonism

**230.** Phencyclidine may best be characterized by which of the following statements?

a. it has opioid activity
b. its mechanism of action is related to its anticholinergic properties
c. it can cause significant hallucinogenic activity
d. it causes significant withdrawal symptoms
e. treatment of overdose is with an opiate

**231.** Which of the following statements about "crack" (the free-base form of cocaine) is true?

a. "flashbacks" (recurrences of effects) may occur months after the last use of the drug
b. it may cause seizures and cardiac arrhythmias
c. it acts by blocking adrenergic receptors
d. it is the salt form of cocaine
e. it is primarily administered intranasally

**DIRECTIONS:** Each numbered question or incomplete statement below is NEGATIVELY phrased. Select the **one best** lettered response.

**232.** All the following compounds are indicated for the treatment of psychoses EXCEPT

a.   perphenazine
b.   thiothixene hydrochloride
c.   fluoxetine hydrochloride
d.   haloperidol
e.   loxapine succinate

**233.** Triazolam, a central nervous system (CNS) depressant, is characterized by all the following statements EXCEPT

a.   it binds to benzodiazepine receptor, enhancing γ-aminobutyric acid (GABA)-mediated chloride (Cl⁻) influx
b.   it is useful in the treatment of insomnia
c.   it enhances the activity of the drug-metabolizing microsomal system
d.   combined with ethanol, it may produce significant respiratory depression
e.   adverse effects may include drowsiness, dizziness, lethargy, and ataxia

**234.** All the statements that follow accurately describe the pharmacology of lidocaine EXCEPT

a.   it acts by interfering with sodium (Na) influx in nerve fibers
b.   coadministration of epinephrine would prolong its duration of action
c.   adverse reactions to its use may include CNS and cardiovascular depression
d.   it is biotransformed by plasma esterases
e.   it is slowly metabolized in the fetus and neonate

**235.** All the following benzodiazepines are biotransformed to active products EXCEPT

a.   alprazolam
b.   diazepam
c.   oxazepam
d.   prazepam
e.   chlordiazepoxide

**236.** Effects of thioridazine include all the following EXCEPT

a.   orthostatic hypotension, constipation, and urinary retention
b.   tardive dyskinesia
c.   hypoprolactinemia
d.   antiemesis
e.   control of psychotic behavior

**237.** Flurazepam has all the following characteristics EXCEPT

a.   classification as a benzodiazepine
b.   primary use as a hypnotic
c.   production of physical dependence
d.   effective production of analgesia
e.   long duration of action (greater than 24 h)

**238.** A high degree of tolerance develops to all the following effects of hydromorphone EXCEPT

a.   euphoria
b.   analgesia
c.   nausea and vomiting
d.   respiratory depression
e.   constipation

**239.** All the following statements about methadone are true EXCEPT

a. it is useful as an analgesic
b. it has greater oral efficacy than morphine
c. it possesses opioid antagonist effects
d. it produces a milder but more protracted withdrawal syndrome than that associated with morphine
e. adverse reactions may include constipation, respiratory depression, and lightheadedness

**240.** Thiopental is used as a general anesthetic. All the following statements characterize its actions EXCEPT

a. it is ultra-short-acting by virtue of redistribution
b. it sensitizes the myocardium to endogenous catecholamines? *ketamine?*
c. it may cause laryngospasm and bronchospasm
d. it is biotransformed to pentobarbital
e. it produces little postanesthetic excitement or vomiting

**241.** All the following are typical toxicities of ethanol EXCEPT

a. it is a hepatotoxic agent
b. it elevates body temperature by peripheral vasoconstriction *(vasodilation)*
c. it suppresses the release of antidiuretic hormone
d. it can lead to gastritis and pancreatitis
e. acute overdose can cause acidosis, hypoglycemia, and elevated intracranial pressure

**242.** Lidocaine, a commonly used local anesthetic, has all the following effects EXCEPT

a. it is biotransformed by amidase
b. vasodilation increases duration of action *epinephrine → vasoconstriction*
c. it has rapid onset of action
d. topical application can produce surface anesthesia
e. it can be used to induce epidural anesthesia

**243.** Phenytoin's activities include all the following EXCEPT

a. it appears to suppress the spread of neuronal discharge from an initiating site adjacent to remote brain areas
b. plasma protein binding is greater than 90%
c. its major use is in the treatment of absence seizures *Valproate/Ethosuximide*
d. its major side effect is ataxia
e. it can cause hyperplasia of the gums

**244.** All the following are characteristics of lithium carbonate EXCEPT that it

a. has a general sedation action similar to that of the phenothiazine derivatives
b. may induce tremors and nephrogenic diabetes insipidus
c. is useful in the treatment of bipolar affective (manic-depressive) disorders
d. has a low therapeutic index, and plasma or serum concentrations must be determined to facilitate safe use of the drug
e. will accumulate in patients who are taking any diuretic that will cause significant $Na^+$ depletion

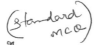

**245.** All the following agents enhance the activity of GABA EXCEPT

a. chlordiazepoxide
b. phenobarbital
c. halazepam
d. valproic acid
e. chlorpromazine

**246.** Marijuana, an addicting drug, has all the following characteristics EXCEPT

a. it may lower intraocular pressure
b. a sign of acute intoxication is reddening of conjunctiva
c. it has antiemetic properties
d. heavy chronic use can lower serum testosterone levels in men
e. it causes flashbacks (LSD)

**247.** All the following drugs produce an abstinence syndrome characterized as being excitatory EXCEPT

a. morphine
b. ethanol
c. phenobarbital
d. cocaine
e. glutethimide

**248.** Naltrexone, a widely used agent in the rehabilitation of opioid-dependent patients, has all the following characteristics EXCEPT

a. it lacks opioid agonist activity at therapeutic doses
b. it possesses longer duration of action than naloxone
c. it will precipitate withdrawal syndrome in a heroin addict
d. it is usually administered IV (oral)
e. it is subject to "first-pass" metabolism in the liver

**249.** Drugs that produce their pharmacologic effects by inhibition of prostaglandin synthesis include all the following EXCEPT

a. indomethacin
b. ibuprofen
c. acetaminophen (don't get confused with aspirin)
d. piroxicam
e. naproxen

**250.** All the following are a consequence of ethanol abuse EXCEPT

a. development of metabolic tolerance
b. reduced effect of barbiturates in an intoxicated alcoholic person
c. possible development of disorientation, tremors, hallucinations, and convulsions when consumption of ethanol is abruptly ended
d. hepatitis
e. pancreatitis

**251.** Barbiturates, in addition to their sedative effects, have all the following characteristics EXCEPT

a. pentobarbital is a biotransformation product of thiopental
b. phenobarbital can decrease the enzymatic activity of δ-aminolevulinic acid
c. mephobarbital can be used in the treatment of tonic-clonic seizures
d. the duration of effect for methohexital is determined by redistribution
e. alkalinization of the urine readily enhances the excretion of secobarbital (forced alkaline diuresis)

*especially for Down's + Pulmonary hypertension* (X)

**252.** Correct statements concerning fentanyl include all the following EXCEPT

a. it has been shown to be up to 100 times more potent than morphine
b. it is usually administered orally
c. it is useful for anesthesia
d. at high doses it produces muscular rigidity, which is reversed by naloxone
e. it is combined with droperidol to produce neuroleptanalgesia

*(read)*

**253.** The general anesthetic halothane has all the following characteristics EXCEPT

a. it is more potent as an anesthetic than nitrous oxide
b. it increases cardiac output *(hypotension)*
c. it causes respiratory depression with increased anesthetic levels
d. it may produce hepatotoxicity
e. it is a halogenated alkane

**254.** The mechanisms of drugs used in the therapy of parkinsonism include all the following EXCEPT

a. benztropine blocks muscarinic receptors
b. amantadine stimulates release of dopamine from storage sites
c. bromocriptine stimulates dopaminergic receptors
d. L-dopa enhances the synthesis of dopamine
e. selegiline is an inhibitor of MAO-A

*(MAO-B)*

**255.** At a follow-up visit one month after a 22-year-old male was newly diagnosed with schizophrenia and started on chlorpromazine, he has several complaints, listed below. Which of them CANNOT be attributed to chlorpromazine?

a. a "restless feeling"
b. sexual dysfunction
c. urinary hesitancy
d. vomiting *(Anti-emetic)*

**256.** A 27-year-old male presents with reactive depression following the accidental death of a close relative. A tricyclic antidepressant is chosen to control his depression. Which adverse effects would NOT be of concern?

a. disturbance in rapid-eye-movement (REM) sleep
b. sedation
c. dry mouth
d. orthostatic hypotension
e. tardive dyskinesia

*Drug classification  Read carefully*

*Anti  depressants*
*Psychotic*

*Influenza A*
*Blocks the entry of Virus (receptor level)*

*Read where are distributed*

**DIRECTIONS:** Each group of questions below consists of lettered headings followed by a set of numbered items. For each numbered item select the one lettered heading with which it is **most** closely associated. Each lettered heading may be used **once, more than once, or not at all.**

## Questions 257–260

For each patient, select the drug of choice:

a. midazolam
b. diazepam
c. alprazolam
d. clonazepam
e. oxazepam

**257.** A 38-year-old male with a 15-year history of grand mal seizures is brought to the ED with generalized tonic-clonic seizures that are unremittent. *Diazepam.*

**258.** A 16-year-old female is brought to the ED by her mother, who has observed that her daughter has abruptly experienced an impairment of consciousness associated with clonic jerking of the eyelids and staring into space lasting approximately 30 seconds.

**259.** A 48-year-old female has had difficulty swallowing for six months. She is premedicated for an endoscopic examination. *Midazolam*

**260.** A 12-year-old boy develops uncontrollable panic while camping with his parents in the Mojave Desert. *alprazolam*

*Benzodiazapines*

## Questions 261–263

Match each description with the appropriate drug.

a. primidone
b. disulfiram
c. dextroamphetamine
d. valproic acid
e. flurazepam
f. phenylephrine
g. phenytoin
h. isoetharine
i. carbamazepine
j. amitriptyline
k. triazolam
l. diazepam

**261.** Causes megaloblastic anemia, ataxia, and gingival hyperplasia *phenytoin*

**262.** Is used in the management of ethanol withdrawal, as a pre-anesthetic medication, and in the treatment of status epilepticus *Diazepam*

**263.** May cause increased alertness, elevated mood states, insomnia, irritability, and hallucinations *Dextroamphetamine*

## Questions 264-266

Many drugs are associated with an ability to induce physical dependence as well as a craving for and tolerance to their psychological effects. For each of the drugs listed below, choose the effect that it usually produces.

a.  psychic dependence
b.  tachyphylaxis
c.  physical dependence only
d.  tolerance and physical dependence
e.  hallucinations
f.  psychedelic effects
g.  low potential of addiction

**264.** Meperidine

**265.** Secobarbital

**266.** Chlorpromazine

**267.** A 19-year-old female whose roommate is being treated for depression decides that she is also depressed and secretly takes her roommate's pills "as directed on the bottle" for several days. One night, she makes herself a snack of chicken liver paté and bleu cheese, accompanied by a glass of red wine. She soon develops headache, nausea, and palpitations. She goes to the ED, where her blood pressure is found to be 200/110 mmHg. What antidepressant did she take?

a.  sertraline
b.  phenelzine
c.  nortriptyline
d.  trazodone
e.  fluoxetine

**268.** A 41-year-old female is seen in the psychiatric clinic for a follow-up appointment. She has been taking an antidepressant for three weeks with some improvement in mood. However, she complains of drowsiness, palpitations, dry mouth, and feeling faint on standing. Which antidepressant is she taking?

a.  amitriptyline
b.  trazodone
c.  fluoxetine
d.  venlafaxine
e.  bupropion

**269.** A 31-year-old female has been treated with fluoxetine for two months with no improvement in her depression. You decide to switch antidepressant therapy to phenelzine and instruct her to wait one week after stopping fluoxetine to start taking the new pills. She does not follow these instructions. Two days later, she is brought to the ED with unstable vital signs, muscle rigidity, myoclonus, and hyperthermia. What caused these findings?

a.  increased serotonin (5-HT) in synapses
b.  increased norepinephrine in synapses
c.  increased acetylcholine in synapses
d.  increased dopamine in synapses

**270.** A 36-year-old male unemployed dishwasher with no history of seizures presents with difficulty thinking coherently and claiming he is an astronaut. Following treatment, he suddenly has a grand mal seizure. Which neuroleptic agent was administered?

a.  haloperidol
b.  fluphenazine
c.  clozapine
d.  molindone
e.  loxapine

**271.** A 31-year-old female is treated with an antipsychotic agent because of a recent history of spontaneously removing her clothing in public places and claiming that she hears voices telling her to do so. Her blood pressure is normally 130/70 mmHg. Since being treated with a drug, she has had several bouts of syncope. Orthostatic hypotension was noted on physical examination. Which drug is most likely to cause this?

a.  haloperidol
b.  molindone
c.  loxapine
d.  thioridazine
e.  pimozide

**272.** A 29-year-old male uses secobarbital to satisfy his addiction to barbiturates. During the past week, he is imprisoned and is not able to obtain the drug. He is brought to the prison medical ward because of the onset of severe anxiety, increased sensitivity to light, dizziness, and generalized tremors. On physical examination, he is hyperreflexic. Which of the following agents should he be given to diminish his withdrawal symptoms?

a.  buspirone
b.  chloral hydrate
c.  chlorpromazine
d.  diazepam
e.  trazodone

**273.** A 72-year-old female with a long history of anxiety treated with diazepam decides to triple her dose because of increasing fearfulness about "environmental noises." Several days after her attempt at self-prescribing, her neighbor finds her to be extremely lethargic and non-responsive. On examination, she is found to be stuporous and have diminished reaction to pain and decreased reflexes. Her respiratory rate is 8 breaths per minute (BPM), and she has shallow respirations. Which antidote could be given to reverse these findings?

a.  naltrexone
b.  physostigmine
c.  pralidoxime
d.  flumazenil

**274.** A 36-year-old male has been experiencing intense pressure to be more productive at work. This has resulted in his becoming extremely anxious, which makes it very difficult for him to function effectively. He wishes to keep his job. Physical examination and blood chemistries are normal. He is given diazepam, which diminishes his anxiety and allows him to concentrate on his work. What is this drug's mechanism of action?

a. it directly opens the Cl⁻ channel of the GABA receptor
b. it increases the frequency of opening of the Cl⁻ channel of the GABA receptor
c. it prolongs the duration of opening of the Cl⁻ channel of the GABA receptor

**275.** A 10-year-old female asthmatic patient receives cromolyn daily as part of her therapeutic regimen. Cromolyn functions primarily as:

a. a $\beta_2$-agonist
b. a histamine$_1$ (H$_1$) receptor antagonist
c. an anticholinergic
d. an inhibitor of mediator release

**276.** A 29-year-old male requires suturing for a deep laceration in his palm. He is allergic to benzocaine. Which of the following local anesthetics could safely be used?

a. cocaine
b. tetracaine
c. bupivacaine
d. procaine

**277.** A 45-year-old male with alcoholic cirrhosis is seen in the ED because of a laceration of the scalp. Of the following local anesthetics, which would potentially be toxic?

a. lidocaine
b. benzocaine
c. procaine
d. tetracaine

**278.** Which best describes the mechanism of interaction of cimetidine with alprazolam?

a. it decreases alprazolam metabolism
b. it decreases alprazolam sensitivity at the site of action
c. it decreases alprazolam renal excretion
d. it decreases alprazolam plasma protein binding
e. it decreases alprazolam intestinal absorption

**279.** Which best describes the mechanism of interaction of nonsteroidal anti-inflammatory drugs (NSAIDs) with lithium salts?

a. they increase lithium intestinal absorption
b. they increase lithium renal reabsorption
c. they increase lithium plasma protein binding
d. they increase lithium sensitivity at its site of action

# CENTRAL NERVOUS SYSTEM

## Answers

**205. The answer is c.** (*Hardman and Limbird, 9/e, p 546.*) Pentazocine is a mixed agonist-antagonist of opioid receptors. When a partial agonist, such as pentazocine, displaces a full agonist, such as methadone, the receptor is less activated; this leads to withdrawal syndrome in an opioid-dependent person.

**206. The answer is c.** (*DiPalma, 4/e, p 327. Hardman and Limbird, 9/e, pp 543–544.*) Fentanyl is a chemical relative of meperidine that is nearly 100 times more potent than morphine. The duration of action, usually between 30 and 60 min after parenteral administration, is shorter than that of meperidine. Fentanyl citrate is only available for parenteral administration intramuscularly and IV. ( Fentanyl - Neat ⇒ standard conc )

**207. The answer is d.** (*DiPalma, 4/e, pp 365–371, 373.*) Local anesthetics are agents that, when applied locally, block nerve conduction; they also prevent generation of a nerve impulse. All contain a lipophilic (benzene) functional group and most a hydrophilic (amine) group. Benzocaine does not contain the terminal hydrophilic amine group; thus, it is only slightly soluble in water and is slowly absorbed with a prolonged duration. It is, therefore, only useful as a surface anesthetic.

**208. The answer is c.** (*DiPalma, 4/e, pp 275–282. Hardman and Limbird, 9/e, pp 414–416.*) Unwanted pharmacologic side effects produced by phenothiazine antipsychotic drugs (e.g., perphenazine) include Parkinson-like syndrome, akathisia, dystonias, galactorrhea, amenorrhea, and infertility. These side effects are due to the ability of these agents to block dopamine receptors. The phenothiazines also block muscarinic and α-adrenergic receptors, which are responsible for other effects.

**209. The answer is d.** (*DiPalma, 4/e, pp 225–226. Hardman and Limbird, 9/e, p 188.*) Malignant hyperthermia (hyperpyrexia), a syndrome associated with use of a general anesthetic (e.g., halothane) in conjunction with a skeletal muscle relaxant, is characterized by tachycardia, hyperventilation, arrhythmias, fever, muscular fasciculation, and rigidity. It is caused by a sudden increase in the availability of calcium (Ca) ions in the myoplasma of muscle. Dantrolene, which interferes with release of Ca ions from the sarcoplasmic reticulum, is indicated in treatment of the disorder. The first three agents are centrally acting skeletal muscle relaxants that are not useful in the treatment of malignant hyperthermia.

**210. The answer is b.** (*DiPalma, 4/e, p 298. Katzung, 7/e, p 1067.*) Fatalities have been reported when fluoxetine and MAO inhibitors (MAOIs) such as tranylcypromine have been given simultaneously. MAOIs should be stopped at least 2 weeks before administration of fluoxetine or paroxetine. The mechanism of this interaction is under investigation.

**211. The answer is c.** (*DiPalma, 4/e, p 290. Hardman and Limbird, 9/e, p 436.*) The tricyclics and second-generation antidepressants act by blocking serotonin or norepinephrine uptake into the presynaptic terminal. Fluoxetine selectively inhibits serotonin uptake with minimal effects on norepinephrine uptake. Protriptyline, maprotiline, desipramine, and amoxapine have greater effect on norepinephrine uptake.

**212. The answer is d.** (*DiPalma, 4/e, pp 224–225. Hardman and Limbird, 9/e, pp 308–313.*) Halothane is a substituted alkane general anesthetic. It undergoes significant metabolism in humans with about 20% of the absorbed dose recovered as metabolites. Halothane can cause postoperative jaundice and hepatic necrosis with repeated administration in rare instances.

**213. The answer is c.** (*DiPalma, 4/e, pp 314–316. Hardman and Limbird, 9/e, p 510.*) Carbidopa is an inhibitor of aromatic L-amino acid decarboxylase. It cannot readily penetrate the CNS and thus decreases the decarboxylation of L-dopa in the peripheral tissues. This promotes an increased concentration of L-dopa in the nigrostriatum, where it is converted to dopamine. In addition, the effective dose of L-dopa can be reduced.

**214. The answer is c.** (*DiPalma, 4/e, p 232. Katzung, 7/e, pp 364–365.*) Flumazenil is a competitive benzodiazepine receptor antagonist. The drug reverses the CNS sedative effects of benzodiazepines and is indicated where general anesthesia has been induced by or maintained with benzodiazepines such as diazepam, lorazepam, or midazolam.

**215. The answer is d.** (*DiPalma, 4/e, pp 319–324. Hardman and Limbird, 9/e, pp 521–522.*) The enkephalins are endogenous agonists of the opioid receptors. They are located in areas of the brain and spinal cord related to the perception of pain. These areas include the laminae I and II of the spinal cord, the spinal trigeminal nucleus, and the periaqueductal gray. Selegiline and trihexyphenidyl are anti-parkinsonism drugs; baclofen is a skeletal muscle relaxant agonist for the GABA receptor.

**216. The answer is b.** (*DiPalma, 4/e, pp 250–251. Hardman and Limbird, 9/e, p 484.*) IV administered diazepam is the drug of choice for treatment of status epilepticus. Diazepam increases the apparent affinity of the inhibitory neurotransmitter GABA for binding sites on brain cell membranes. The effects of diazepam are short-lasting. Continuing therapy is usually with phenytoin. Other drugs suggested for use in status epilepticus are lorazepam and lidocaine. None of the other drugs listed in the question are appropriate for status epilepticus: chlorpromazine is an antipsychotic; succinylcholine is a neuromuscular blocking agent; tranylcypromine is an antidepressant; ethosuximide is used in petit mal epilepsy.

**217. The answer is a.** (*DiPalma, 4/e, pp 294–296. Hardman and Limbird, 9/e, p 436.*) The most common side effects associated with antidepressants are their antimuscarinic effects, which may be evident in over 50% of patients. Clinically, the antimuscarinic effects may manifest as dry mouth, blurred vision, constipation, tachycardia, dizziness, and urinary retention. At therapeutic plasma concentrations these drugs usually do not cause changes in the EKG. Direct cardiac effects of the tricyclic antidepressants are important in overdosage.

**218. The answer is c.** (*Hardman and Limbird, 9/e, pp 632–633.*) Nausea, vomiting, abdominal pain, and diarrhea are early signs of the severe liver toxicity caused by high levels of acetaminophen; other symptoms of acetaminophen toxicity include dizziness, excitement, and disorientation. N-acetylcysteine is the appropriate treatment for acetaminophen overdose.

**219. The answer is c.** (*DiPalma, 4/e, pp 315–318. Katzung, 7/e, pp 484–485.*) Two types of MAO have been found: MAO-A, which metabolizes norepinephrine and serotonin, and MAO-B, which metabolizes dopamine. Deprenyl (selegiline) is a selective inhibitor of MAO-B. It therefore inhibits the breakdown of dopamine and prolongs the therapeutic effectiveness of L-dopa in parkinsonism. Bromocriptine is a dopamine receptor agonist. Carbidopa inhibits the peripheral metabolism of L-dopa. Both are useful in treatment of parkinsonism. Phenelzine and tranylcypromine are nonselective MAOIs. Combining them with L-dopa may lead to hypertensive crises, and thus they are not used in the therapy of parkinsonism.

**220. The answer is c.** (*DiPalma, 4/e, pp 375–378. Hardman and Limbird, 9/e, pp 556–559.*) In opioid abuse, there is always a high degree of cross tolerance to other drugs with a similar pharmacologic action even if the chemical composition of the opioids is totally different. Tolerance develops at different rates to different effects of opioids. With methadone, abrupt withdrawal causes a syndrome that is qualitatively similar to that of morphine but is longer and less intense, thus following the general rule that a drug with a shorter duration of action produces a shorter, more intense withdrawal syndrome. The crimes associated with narcotic abuse are considered to be motivated by the need to acquire the drug and not from the effects of the drug per se. Significant tolerance develops to most of the effects of narcotics except for constipation and pinpoint pupils, to which there is minimal tolerance.

**221. The answer is c.** (*Hardman and Limbird, 9/e, p 527. Katzung, 7/e, p 502.*) Naloxone is a pure opioid antagonist at the μ, κ, and δ receptors. μ-receptor stimulation causes analgesia, euphoria, decreased gastrointestinal (GI) activity, miosis, and respiratory depression. κ-receptor stimulation causes analgesia, dysphoria, and psychotomimetic effects. δ-receptor stimulation is not fully understood in humans, but is associated with analgesia and antinociception for thermal stimuli.

**222. The answer is b.** (*DiPalma, 4/e, p 318. Hardman and Limbird, 9/e, p 451.*) Selegiline inhibits MAO-B, thus delaying the metabolic breakdown of dopamine. It is effective alone in parkinsonism and increases the effectiveness of L-dopa. Benztropine and trihexyphenidyl are cholinergic antagonists in the brain; bromocriptine is a dopamine receptor agonist. Chlorpromazine is an antipsychotic drug with antiadrenergic properties.

**223. The answer is b.** (*DiPalma, 4/e, pp 317–318. Katzung, 7/e, pp 455–456.*) Bromocriptine mimics the action of dopamine in the brain but is not as readily metabolized. It is especially useful in parkinsonism that is unresponsive to L-dopa. Apomorphine is also a dopamine receptor agonist, but its side effects preclude its use for this purpose. Selegiline is an MAO-B inhibitor, atropine is a belladonna preparation, and amantadine is an antiviral agent that probably affects the synthesis or uptake of dopamine.

**224. The answer is a.** (*DiPalma, 4/e, pp 275–277. Isselbacher, 13/e, pp 2417–2418.*) Chlorpromazine is the prototype compound of the phenothiazine class of antipsychotic drugs. It is indicated for use in the treatment of a variety of psychoses, which includes schizophrenia, and in the treatment of nausea and vomiting, in both adults and children, from a number of causes. The drug can be administered orally, rectally, or intramuscularly for this purpose. It is believed that the effectiveness of the compound is based on inhibition of dopaminergic receptors in the chemoreceptor trigger zone of the medulla. Other phenothiazine derivatives are also used for emesis, including thiethylperazine, prochlorperazine, and perphenazine. Although chlorpromazine may cause orthostatic hypotension and has mild $H_1$-histamine receptor blocking activity, the drug is never used as an antihypertensive or as an antihistaminic. Chlorpromazine is not an effective antidepressant drug and lithium salts are used for treating the mania associated with bipolar affective disorder.

**225. The answer is c.** (*DiPalma, 4/e, pp 325–333. Hardman and Limbird, 9/e, pp 528–537.*) Morphine is a pure agonist opioid drug with agonist activity toward all the opioid subtype receptor sites. In high doses, deaths associated with morphine are related to the depression of the respiratory center in the medulla. Morphine has a high addiction potential related to the activity of heroin or dihydromorphine. Codeine has a significantly lower addiction potential.

**226. The answer is d.** (*DiPalma, 4/e, pp 269–270. Hardman and Limbird, 9/e, pp 338, 570.*) Cocaine has local anesthetic properties; it can block the initiation or conduction of a nerve impulse. It is biotransformed by plasma esterases to inactive products. In addition, cocaine blocks the reuptake of norepinephrine. This action produces CNS stimulant effects including euphoria, excitement, and restlessness. Peripherally, cocaine produces sympathomimetic effects including tachycardia and vasoconstriction. Death from acute overdose can be from respiratory depression or cardiac failure. Cocaine is an ester of benzoic acid and closely related to the structure of atropine.

Dopamine → Prolactin Inhibiting factor

**227. The answer is b.** (*DiPalma, 4/e, pp 275–277, 317. Hardman and Limbird, 9/e, p 282–283.*) Central dopamine receptors are divided into $D_1$ and $D_2$ receptors. Antipsychotic activity is better correlated to blockade of $D_2$ receptors. Haloperidol, a potent antipsychotic, selectively antagonizes at $D_2$ receptors. Phenothiazine derivatives, such as chlorpromazine, fluphenazine, and promethazine, are not selective for $D_2$ receptors. Bromocriptine, a selective $D_2$ agonist, is useful in the treatment of parkinsonism and hyperprolactinemia. It produces fewer adverse reactions than do nonselective dopamine receptor agonists.

**228. The answer is d.** (*DiPalma, 4/e, p 283. Hardman and Limbird, 9/e, pp 407–412.*) Haloperidol is a butyrophenone derivative with the same mechanism of action as the phenothiazines, that is, blockade of dopaminergic receptors. It is more selective for $D_2$ receptors. Haloperidol is more potent on a weight basis than the phenothiazines, but produces a higher incidence of extrapyramidal reactions than does chlorpromazine.

**229. The answer is c.** (*Hardman and Limbird, 9/e, pp 415–416.*) NMS is thought to be a severe form of an extrapyramidal syndrome that can occur at any time with any dose of a neuroleptic agent. However, the risk is higher when high-potency agents are used in high doses, especially if given parenterally. Mortality from NMS is greater than 10%.

**230. The answer is c.** (*DiPalma, 4/e, pp 381–382. Hardman and Limbird, 9/e, pp 574–575.*) Phencyclidine is a hallucinogenic compound with no opioid activity. Its mechanism of action is amphetamine-like. A withdrawal syndrome has not been described for this drug in human subjects. In overdose the treatment of choice for the psychotic activity is the antipsychotic drug haloperidol.

Drug of choice → haloperidol

**231. The answer is b.** (*DiPalma, 4/e, pp 380–381. Katzung, 7/e, p 522.*) "Crack" is the free-base (nonsalt) form of the alkaloid cocaine. It is called crack because when heated it makes a crackling sound. Heating crack enables a person to smoke it; the drug is readily absorbed through the lungs and produces an intense euphoric effect in seconds. Use has led to seizures and cardiac arrhythmias. Some of cocaine's effects (sympathomimetic) are due to blockade of norepinephrine reuptake into presynaptic terminals; it does not block receptors. "Flashbacks" can occur with use of LSD and mescaline but have not been associated with the use of cocaine.

*classification*
*(ATC)*

**232. The answer is c.** (*DiPalma, 4/e, pp 275–286. Hardman and Limbird, 9/e, pp 404–406.*) There are several chemical classes of compounds useful as antipsychotic agents. Phenothiazine derivatives (e.g., perphenazine) constitute the most numerous group and were the first antipsychotic drugs to be used. Thiothixene hydrochloride and chlorprothixene are two thiothixene derivatives used as antipsychotic drugs; butyrophenone derivatives are exemplified by haloperidol. Several other classes of heterocyclic compounds have antipsychotic activity, including loxapine succinate, molindone hydrochloride, and pimozide. Fluoxetine hydrochloride is used as an antidepressant; it has no significant antipsychotic activity.

**233. The answer is c.** (*DiPalma, 4/e, pp 244–248. Katzung, 7/e, p 373.*) Triazolam is a benzodiazepine derivative, and like flurazepam and temazepam it is useful in the treatment of insomnia. It acts by binding to benzodiazepine receptors, enhancing GABA-mediated Cl⁻ influx. Adverse reactions include drowsiness, dizziness, lethargy, and ataxia. Though benzodiazepines alone do not significantly depress respiration, in combination with ethanol they can lead to severe respiratory depression. Unlike the barbiturates, benzodiazepines do not significantly induce the drug-metabolizing microsomal system at therapeutic doses.

*(MCQ → Based on This)*

**234. The answer is d.** (*DiPalma, 4/e, pp 365–374.*) Lidocaine is an amide-type local anesthetic. It acts by interfering with influx of Na into nerve fibers. Lidocaine is biotransformed in the liver; being an amide, it is not hydrolyzed by plasma esterases. Coadministration of epinephrine causes local vasoconstriction, thus prolonging the duration of action. Adverse reactions caused by plasma buildup include CNS excitation followed by depression and cardiovascular depression.

**235. The answer is c.** (*DiPalma, 4/e, pp 247–248. Hardman and Limbird, 9/e, pp 423–424.*) Some benzodiazepines are biotransformed to active products with CNS effects, some of which are long-lived. Desmethyldiazepam is a long-acting metabolite of chlordiazepoxide, clorazepate, alprazolam, diazepam, and prazepam. These compounds are more likely to produce cumulative effects and residual effects such as excessive drowsiness. Oxazepam and lorazepam are biotransformed to the inactive glucuronide.

**236. The answer is c.** (*DiPalma, 4/e, pp 280–282. Hardman and Limbird, 9/e, pp 414–416.*) The phenothiazines (e.g., thioridazine) are antipsychotic

*(That's why used in BAPLS guidelines of status epilepticus)*

agents. Autonomic manifestations result from α-adrenergic receptor and muscarinic cholinergic receptor blockade. A Parkinson-like syndrome results from blockade of dopaminergic receptors in the basal ganglia. Thioridazine has a lower incidence of acute extrapyramidal reactions than higher potency agents such as haloperidol and trifluoperazine. Chronic use of all these agents often leads to tardive dyskinesia. Although effective against vomiting produced by some drugs and disease states, phenothiazines are not effective for control of motion sickness. The phenothiazines block dopaminergic receptors in the pituitary, which subsequently increases secretion of prolactin, causing hyperprolactinemia and galactorrhea.

**237. The answer is d.** (*DiPalma, 4/e, pp 238–239. Hardman and Limbird, 9/e, pp 372–373.*) Estazolam, flurazepam, quazepam, temazepam, and triazolam are all benzodiazepine derivatives that are used exclusively for their hypnotic effect. Flurazepam can cause physical dependence but does not have analgesic properties. It undergoes an *N*-dealkylation reaction to yield *N*-desalkylflurazepam, which has an elimination half-life of 76 to 160 h.

**238. The answer is e.** (*DiPalma, 4/e, pp 331–332. Hardman and Limbird, 9/e, pp 528–537.*) The extent and rate at which tolerance develops to the effects of opioid analgesics vary. A high degree of tolerance develops to analgesia, euphoria, sedation, respiratory depression, antidiuresis, nausea and vomiting, and cough suppression. A moderate degree develops to bradycardia. Little or no tolerance develops to the drug-induced miosis, constipation, and convulsions.

**239. The answer is c.** (*DiPalma, 4/e, pp 337–338. Hardman and Limbird, 9/e, pp 544–545.*) Methadone is an opioid receptor agonist. It is used as an analgesic and to treat opioid abstinence and heroin users (methadone maintenance). The drug has greater oral efficacy than morphine and a much longer biologic half-life; this accounts for the milder but more protracted abstinence syndrome associated with methadone. Methadone does not possess opioid antagonist properties and thus would not precipitate withdrawal symptoms in a heroin addict, as would naloxone or naltrexone.

**240. The answer is b.** (*DiPalma, 4/e, pp 228–229. Hardman and Limbird, 9/e, pp 321–323.*) Thiopental is an IV general anesthetic. It is very useful for short procedures because it produces a rapid recovery, which is due to redistribution out of the brain. It produces little postanesthetic excitement or vomiting. Thiopental is biotransformed in the liver by desulfuration to pentobarbital. The compound can produce cough, laryngospasm, and bronchospasm. Thiopental, unlike halothane and related inhalation anesthetics, does *not* sensitize the myocardium to endogenous catecholamines.

**241. The answer is b.** *(DiPalma, 4/e, pp 253–259. Hardman and Limbird, 9/e, pp 386–393.)* Ethanol is a CNS depressant. Among its many effects, it suppresses the release of antidiuretic hormone. Ethanol also causes peripheral vasodilation, particularly of cutaneous blood vessels. Though this may give one a feeling of warmth, heat is being dissipated and body temperature is lowered. Chronic use can lead to gastritis, pancreatitis, cirrhosis of the liver, and central effects such as Wernicke's encephalopathy and Korsakoff's psychosis. Acute overdose can lead to acidosis, hypoglycemia, and elevated intracranial pressure.

**242. The answer is b.** *(DiPalma, 4/e, pp 365–374. Hardman and Limbird, 9/e, pp 338–339.)* Lidocaine is classified as an amide local anesthetic agent and has a rapid onset of action and excellent potency. It is a versatile agent useful in many clinical applications, such as surface anesthesia, peripheral nerve block, infiltration, and spinal and epidural anesthesia. Lidocaine may be combined with epinephrine to increase the former's duration of action. The vasoconstrictor effect of epinephrine will reduce the removal of lidocaine from its site of action. Lidocaine is biotransformed in the liver by amidases and undergoes *N*-dealkylation followed by sulfate conjugation.

**243. The answer is c.** *(DiPalma, 4/e, pp 306–309. Hardman and Limbird, 9/e, pp 468–470.)* Phenytoin's mechanism of action is based on curtailing the capacity of neurons to fire at very high frequencies. Plasma protein binding is approximately 90% in patients with normal amounts of circulating plasma proteins. The major clinical use is in the treatment of tonic-clonic seizures that are or become generalized complex partial seizures. The drug is not useful in absence seizures. The most common dose-related toxicity is a motor disturbance such as ataxia. Although rare, hyperplasia of the gums may occur.

**244. The answer is a.** *(DiPalma, 4/e, pp 286–288. Hardman and Limbird, 9/e, pp 446–449.)* Lithium salts, such as lithium carbonate and lithium citrate, help to prevent the mania and to control mood swings in manic-depressive disorders. Unlike the phenothiazine derivatives, lithium is not a sedative; tremor is one of the most frequent adverse effects of lithium treatment. Renal toxicity includes lithium-induced nephrogenic diabetes insipidus and chronic interstitial nephritis during long-term therapy. Lithium also reduces thyroid function and produces edema. However, the use of diuretics to treat the lithium-induced edema will reduce the Na$^+$ concentrations in the body, which will promote the retention of lithium, thus increasing the potential toxicity of the drug. Since the safe and effective plasma concentration is considered to be between 0.75 and 1.25 meq/L, and concentrations above 2 meq/L have been associated with increased risk of more severe toxicity, the plasma concentrations of lithium should be monitored regularly.

**245. The answer is e.** (*DiPalma, 4/e, pp 244-245, 254–256. Hardman and Limbird, 9/e, pp 280–281.*) GABA is an inhibitory neurotransmitter that activates the Cl$^-$ channel. Benzodiazepines (e.g., chlordiazepoxide, halazepam) bind to receptors on the Cl$^-$ channel and enhance the binding of GABA to its receptor. Barbiturates also act on the chloride channel to increase the frequency of opening of the channel. Valproic acid elevates brain levels of GABA by inhibiting GABA metabolism. Chlorpromazine blocks the activity of dopamine receptors and has little or no effect on the GABA system.

**246. The answer is e.** (*DiPalma, 4/e, pp 250–253, 270–274. Hardman and Limbird, 9/e, pp 572–573.*) The active ingredient in marijuana is Δ$^9$-tetrahydrocannabinol. In general, marijuana is a CNS stimulant causing tachycardia, giddiness, and, at high doses, visual hallucinations. Acute intoxication is characterized by reddening of the conjunctiva (bloodshot eyes) owing to local vasodilation. Potential therapeutic uses include antiemesis in cancer chemotherapy and reduction of intraocular pressure in glaucoma. Chronic use has been associated with an "amotivational syndrome" and with a reduction in serum testosterone and sperm count. Flashbacks are a major symptom of use of LSD.

**247. The answer is d.** (*DiPalma, 4/e, pp 375–384. Hardman and Limbird, 9/e, pp 561–562.*) Physical dependence occurs following prolonged use of morphine, ethanol, barbiturates, and nonbarbiturates such as glutethimide. Acute withdrawal of these substances produces an abstinence syndrome, the severity of which depends upon the drug.

*(opposite effect of the Drug)*

Withdrawal of cocaine after chronic use can lead to craving for the drug, prolonged sleep, general fatigue, lassitude, hyperphagia, and depression. This meets the criteria for a withdrawal syndrome.

**248. The answer is d.** *(DiPalma, 4/e, pp 324, 342–343. Hardman and Limbird, 9/e, pp 549–550.)* Naltrexone and naloxone are pure opioid antagonists with no agonist activity at therapeutic doses. In opioid-dependent persons, these agents will precipitate withdrawal syndrome. Naltrexone is much better absorbed from the GI tract and is useful by oral administration. It also has a much longer duration of action, making it useful in treatment programs for drug addicts. Although naltrexone does have a "first-pass" effect in the liver, the metabolic product is also active.

**249. The answer is c.** *(DiPalma, 4/e, pp 345–363. Hardman and Limbird, 9/e, pp 617–642.)* All the drugs mentioned with the exception of acetaminophen achieve their therapeutic and toxic effects by inhibition of prostaglandin synthesis. Known as NSAIDs, the group includes salicylates as well as sulindac and fenoprofen. Acetaminophen is equal in analgesic potency to NSAIDS, but has no effect on prostaglandins. It is also non-ulcerogenic—a great advantage in patients who are ulcer-prone.

**250. The answer is b.** *(DiPalma, 4/e, pp 257–258. Hardman and Limbird, 9/e, pp 386–393.)* Chronic consumption of ethanol causes hypertrophy of the hepatic smooth endoplasmic reticulum with a resultant increase in metabolic enzymes. The induction of the microsomal system may play a role in the enhanced biotransformation of ethanol and, thus, the development of metabolic or dispositional tolerance. Barbiturates are biotransformed via the microsomal system; however, in the presence of ethanol, which is preferentially metabolized, barbiturates remain active longer. Symptoms of ethanol withdrawal can include restlessness, insomnia, tremors, disorientation, hallucinations, and convulsions. Chronic effects of ethanol abuse may include gastritis, pancreatitis, hepatitis, cirrhosis of the liver, and cardiomegaly.

**251. The answer is b.** *(DiPalma, 4/e, pp 233–238. Hardman and Limbird, 9/e, pp 321–323, 390–391, 562–563.)* The termination of the action of ultra-short-acting barbiturates such as methohexital and thiopental is due to redistribution of the drugs from the brain. Following redistribution thiopental is biotransformed to pentobarbital, which is further oxidized to inactive products. Chronic administration of barbiturates can induce enzymes in the liver. Barbiturates are contraindicated in acute intermittent porphyria because they increase δ-aminolevulinic acid, which produces an elevation of porphyrins in the body. In patients with acute intermittent porphyria, the precipitous increase of porphyrins may result in paralysis and death. All barbiturates possess anticonvulsant activity, but only phenobarbital, mephobarbital, and metharbital have antiepileptic properties. These drugs may be used in the treatment of tonic-clonic seizures, psychomotor seizures, and other types of epilepsy. Although alkalinization of the urine may promote the excretion of weak acidic drugs such as the barbiturates, it appears that only the excretion of phenobarbital is enhanced by increasing the pH of the urine. In the renal tubular fluid phenobarbital is converted more to the anionic form, and this form of phenobarbital is not readily reabsorbed by the renal tubular cells.

**252. The answer is b.** (*DiPalma, 4/e, pp 230–231. Hardman and Limbird, 9/e, pp 543–544.*) The synthetic opioid fentanyl is 80 to 100 times more potent than morphine and has a major use in anesthesia. It is combined with droperidol, an antipsychotic butyrophenone, to produce neuroleptanalgesia. Muscular rigidity produced by fentanyl very likely results from opioid influence on dopaminergic transmission in the striatum, an influence that is antagonized by naloxone. Fentanyl is only available as an injection to be used IV in anesthesia.

**253. The answer is b.** (*DiPalma, 4/e, pp 220, 224–226. Hardman and Limbird, 9/e, pp 308–313.*) The high solubility of halothane, a halogenated alkane, in blood and fat allows for the maintenance of anesthetic blood levels for prolonged periods. The death rate associated with halothane is similar to or slightly lower than that of other anesthetic agents. Halothane is a very potent anesthetic (MAC = 0.77) compared with nitrous oxide (MAC = 110). Hepatotoxicity does occasionally occur and appears to increase in incidence with increased exposure to halothane. Depression of respiratory centers expressed as a decreased ventilatory response to carbon dioxide occurs as anesthetic depth increases. Arterial hypotension and a reduction in cardiac output, peripheral resistance, and myocardial contractility occur at surgical levels of anesthesia.

**254. The answer is e.** (*DiPalma, 4/e, pp 314–318. Hardman and Limbird, 9/e, pp 509–513.*) Drugs useful in the therapy of parkinsonism act through several mechanisms. L-dopa, primary therapy for parkinsonism, is the immediate precursor to dopamine and thus increases brain levels of dopamine by enhancing its synthesis. Benztropine is one of several muscarinic blocking agents and is a useful adjunct in therapy. Amantadine, an antiviral agent, acts by stimulating release of dopamine from storage sites. Bromocriptine is a direct agonist at dopaminergic receptors. Selegiline, a relatively new drug, selectively inhibits MOA-B, which is present in the brain. MOA-A is located mainly in the liver and the gut.

**255. The answer is d.** (*Hardman and Limbird, 9/e, p 414.*) Antipsychotic agents, particularly prochlorperazine, are also useful as antiemetic agents, thought to be due to dopamine blockade at the stomach and at the chemoreceptor trigger zone of the medulla.

**256. The answer is e.** (*Hardman and Limbird, 9/e, pp 442–443, 415.*) Tardive dyskinesia is an adverse effect of neuroleptic, not tricyclic, antidepressants.

**257. The answer is b.** (*Hardman and Limbird, 9/e, p 484. Katzung, 7/e, p 405.*) IV diazepam given immediately is highly effective in controlling status epilepticus.

**258. The answer is d.** (*Katzung, 7/e, p 402.*) Clonazepam is very effective in "absence seizures."

**259. The answer is a.** (*Hardman and Limbird, 9/e, p 373. Katzung, 7/e, pp 420–421.*) Midazolam is useful for sedation because it produces a higher incidence of amnesia and has a more rapid onset of action and a shorter half-life than other benzodiazepines used in anesthesia.

**260. The answer is c.** (*Hardman and Limbird 9/e, p 372. Katzung, 7/e, p 365.*) Compared with other benzodiazepines, alprazolam is selective for treating agoraphobia and panic disorders.

**261–263. The answers are 261-g, 262-l, 263-c.** (*DiPalma, 4/e, pp 244–251, 268–269, 303–314. Hardman and Limbird, 9/e, pp 219–221, 372, 469–470.*) Phenytoin is one of the most commonly used antiepileptic agents. Chronic administration has been reported to cause such adverse reactions as ataxia, dizziness, nystagmus, gingival hyperplasia, hirsutism, and megaloblastic anemia.

Diazepam is a benzodiazepine derivative and is effective in management of anxiety, as a preanesthetic medication, in alcohol withdrawal, as a skeletal muscle relaxant, and in seizure disorders. It is useful in status epilepticus, which may occur on withdrawal from a barbiturate. The agent is well absorbed orally, is highly protein-bound (greater than 90%), and is biotransformed in the liver to active products. Flurazepam and triazolam are benzodiazepine derivatives that are used exclusively as hypnotics.

Dextroamphetamine, a mixed-acting adrenergic drug, is more potent than the *l* isomer in producing CNS stimulation. Some CNS effects of use of dextroamphetamine may be increased alertness, elevated mood states, insomnia, irritability, dizziness, violent behavior, and hallucination. Although phenylephrine is an adrenergic agonist, its central stimulatory effects are minimal.

**264–266. The answers are 264-d, 265-d, 266-g.** (*DiPalma, 4/e, pp 233–238, 275–284, 376–378, 381–382.*) Heroin and other opioids (such as morphine and meperidine) exhibit a high degree of tolerance and physical dependence. The magnitudes of rates of tolerance to all the effects of opioids are not necessarily the same. The physical dependence is quite clear from the character and severity of withdrawal symptoms, which include vomiting spasms, abdominal cramps, diarrhea, and acid-base imbalances among others.

Secobarbital exhibits the same pharmacologic properties as other members of the barbiturate class. While there may be considerable tolerance to the sedative and intoxicating effects of the drug, the lethal dose is not much greater in addicted than normal persons. Severe withdrawal symptoms in epileptic patients may include grand mal seizures and delirium.

No current evidence exists that chlorpromazine, an antipsychotic agent, is addicting. Although some tolerance and physical dependence have been suggested, the failure to detect any electroencephalogram (EEG) changes upon abrupt cessation of the drug implies that these effects are not of major importance.

None of these drugs have significant association with hallucinations or psychedelic effects. LSD is the primary agent deemed to possess these attributes.

**267. The answer is b.** (*Hardman and Limbird, 9/e, p 444.*) This patient ate tyramine-rich foods while taking an MAOI and went into hypertensive crisis. Tyramine causes release of stored catecholamines from presynaptic terminals, which can cause hypertension, headache, tachycardia, cardiac arrhythmias, nausea, and stroke. In patients who do not take MAOIs, tyramine is inactivated in the gut by MAO, and patients taking MAOIs must be warned about the dangers of eating tyramine-rich foods.

**268. The answer is a.** *(Katzung, 7/e, p 493.)* Of the listed antidepressants, only amitriptyline, a tricyclic, causes adverse effects related to blockade of muscarinic acetylcholine receptors. Both trazodone and amitriptyline cause adverse effects related to α-adrenoreceptor blockade.

**269. The answer is a.** *(Hardman and Limbird, 9/e, p 444.)* This patient has the serotonin syndrome. Serotonin is already present in increased amounts in synapses because of blockade of its reuptake by the selective serotonin reuptake inhibitors (SSRI). The amount of serotonin present is further increased when breakdown by MAO is inhibited. The serotonin syndrome can be life threatening.

**270. The answer is c.** *(Hardman and Limbird, 9/e, p 408.)* Clozapine differs from other neuroleptic agents in that it can induce seizures in nonepileptic patients. In patients with a history of epileptic seizures for which they are not receiving treatment, stimulation of seizures can occur following administration of neuroleptic agents because they lower seizure threshold and cause brain discharge patterns reminiscent of epileptic seizure disorders.

**271. The answer is d.** *(Hardman and Limbird, 9/e, pp 404–406.)* Although most antipsychotic agents can cause orthostatic hypotension, thioridazine is the most likely choice of the agents above for causing this adverse effect.

**272. The answer is d.** *(Hardman and Limbird, 9/e, p 564.)* A long-acting benzodiazepine, such as diazepam, is effective in blocking the secobarbital withdrawal symptoms. The anxiolytic effects of buspirone take several days to develop, obviating its use for acute severe anxiety.

**273. The answer is d.** *(Hardman and Limbird, 9/e, p 564. Katzung, 7/e, pp 363, 980.)* Flumazenil is a competitive antagonist of benzodiazepines at the γ-aminobutyric acid (GABA) receptor. Repeated administration is necessary because of its short half-life relative to that of most benzodiazepines.

**274. The answer is b.** (*Hardman and Limbird, 9/e, pp 365–367.*) Benzodiazepines, such as diazepam, bind to the GABA receptor/ion channel complex, enhancing GABA-induced Cl⁻ currents related to more frequent bursts of Cl⁻ channel opening by GABA.

**275. The answer is d.** (*DiPalma, 4/e, pp 489–490. Hardman and Limbird, 9/e, pp 668–669.*) Cromolyn inhibits the release of mediators from mast cells, including histamine and slow-reacting substance of anaphylaxis (SRS-A), which prevents allergically induced bronchospasm. Cromolyn is of no use in an acute asthmatic attack, but is of considerable help in asthma prophylaxis, particularly in children.

**276. The answer is c.** (*Hardman and Limbird, 9/e, p 340. Katzung, 7/e, p 426.*) Of the listed agents, only bupivacaine is an amide. Allergy to amide-type local anesthetics is much less frequent than with ester-type local anesthetics, such as benzocaine; patients who demonstrate allergy to one such drug will be allergic to all of them.

**277. The answer is a.** (*Hardman and Limbird, 9/e, p 338. Katzung, 7/e, p 427.*) Ester-type local anesthetics are mainly hydrolyzed by pseudocholinesterases. Amide-type local anesthetics are hydrolyzed by microsomal enzymes in the liver. Of the listed agents, only lidocaine is an amide and can be influenced by liver dysfunction.

**278. The answer is a.** (*Hardman and Limbird, 9/e, p 906. Katzung, 7/e, pp 1064–1065.*) Cimetidine inhibits the activity of cytochrome P-450, slowing alprazolam metabolism.

**279. The answer is b.** (*Hardman and Limbird, 9/e, p 448. Katzung, 7/e, pp 478, 1067.*) Some NSAIDs can increase proximal tubular reabsorption of lithium salts, which can create toxic levels of lithium in the plasma.

# AUTONOMIC NERVOUS SYSTEM (Physiology rev.)

**Note: In the classification of drugs, prototype drugs are marked with an asterisk (*).**

General Considerations
  Anatomic
  Physiologic
  Nature of synaptic transmission
  Cholinergic transmission
  Adrenergic transmission
  Receptors, adrenergic and
    cholinergic
Adrenergic Drugs
  Sites and mode of action
  Chemistry and structure-
    activity relationships
  Direct-acting agonists
    Epinephrine*
    Norepinephrine (NE)*
    Isoproterenol*
    Phenylephrine
    Dobutamine
    Salmeterol
    Terbutaline
    Albuterol*
    Pirbuterol
    Bitolterol
    Metaproterenol
    Isoetharine
    Ritodrine
    Tetrahydrozoline
  Indirect-acting agents
    Tyramine*
  Mixed-acting agents

Dopamine (DM)*
Ephedrine*
Phenylpropanolamine
Amphetamines
Pseudoephedrine
Metaraminol
β-Adrenergic Blocking Drugs
  Propranolol*
  Acebutolol
  Atenolol
  Betaxolol
  Bisoprolol
  Carteolol
  Esmolol
  Labetalol
  Metoprolol
  Nadolol
  Penbutolol
  Pindolol
  Sotalol
  Timolol
α-Adrenergic Blocking Drugs
  Nonselective
    Phentolamine*
    Phenoxybenzamine*
  Selective
    Prazosin,* terazosin, doxazosin
    Yohimbine
Adrenergic Neuronal Blocking Drugs
  Reserpine*

Guanethidine,* guanadrel
Metyrosine
Cholinomimetic Agents
Direct-acting
  Choline esters
    Acetylcholine (Ach)*
    Methacholine
    Carbachol
    Bethanechol
  Naturally occurring muscarinic
    alkaloids
    Muscarine*
    Pilocarpine*
  Naturally occurring nicotinic
    alkaloids                    (f(and))
    Nicotine*
    Lobeline
Indirect Acting
  Reversible cholinesterase
    inhibitors
    Physostigmine*
    Neostigmine
    Pyridostigmine
    Edrophonium
    Ambenonium chloride
    Tacrine
      (tetrahydroaminoacridine)
  Irreversible cholinesterase
    inhibitors
    Isoflurophate*
    Echothiophate iodide
    Malathion*
    Soman, sarin, tabun
Antidotes for Organophosphate
  Poisoning
  Atropine
  Pralidoxime chloride
Antimuscarinic Drugs
  Atropine*
  Homatropine*

Scopolamine*
Propantheline bromide
Cyclopentolate
Tropicamide
Dicyclomine
Ipratropium
Methscopolamine
Trihexyphenidyl*
Ganglionic Blocking Drugs
Mecamylamine
Trimethaphan camsylate
Nicotine
Skeletal-Muscle Relaxants
Neuromuscular blocking agents
  Depolarizing drugs
    Succinylcholine*
  Nondepolarizing drugs
    Tubocurarine*
    Metocurine
    Gallamine
    Doxacurium
    Mivacurium
    Pipecuronium
    Pancuronium
    Vecuronium
    Atracurium
Centrally acting skeletal-muscle
  relaxants
  Baclofen
  Cyclobenzaprine
  Diazepam
Direct-acting skeletal-muscle
  relaxant
  Dantrolene
Monoamine Oxidase Inhibitors
  (MAOIs)
  Deprenyl (Selegiline)*
  Tranylcypromine
  Phenelzine

# Questions

**DIRECTIONS:** Each question below contains several suggested responses. Select the **one best** response to each question.

**280.** Of the many types of adrenergic receptors found throughout the body, which is most likely responsible for the cardiac stimulation observed following an intravenous (IV) injection of epinephrine?

a. $\alpha_1$-adrenergic receptors
b. $\alpha_2$-adrenergic receptors
c. $\beta_1$-adrenergic receptors
d. $\beta_2$-adrenergic receptors
e. $\beta_3$-adrenergic receptors

**281.** The enzyme that is inhibited by echothiophate iodide is

a. tyrosine hydroxylase
b. acetylcholinesterase (AchE)
c. catechol-O-methyltransferase (COMT)
d. MAO
e. carbonic anhydrase

**282.** Applied to the skin in a transdermal patch (transdermal therapeutic delivery system), this drug is used to prevent or reduce the occurrence of nausea and vomiting associated with motion sickness.

a. diphenhydramine
b. chlorpromazine
c. ondansetron
d. dimenhydrinate
e. scopolamine

*Anti emetic*

**283.** The nonselective $\beta$-adrenergic blocking agent that is also a competitive antagonist at $\alpha_1$-adrenoceptors is

a. timolol
b. nadolol
c. pindolol
d. acebutolol
e. labetalol

*β Blockade dextrojration m so*

**284.** The contractile effect of various doses of norepinephrine (NE) (X) alone on vascular smooth muscle is represented in the figure below.

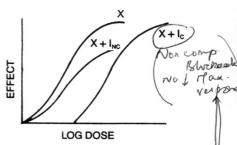

*X + I_C*
*Non comp Blockade*
*no ↓ of max. response*

When combined with an antagonist ($I_C$ or $I_{NC}$), a shift in the dose-response curve occurs. The curve labeled $X + I_{NC}$ would most likely occur when vascular smooth muscle is treated with NE in the presence of

a. terazosin
b. phentolamine
c. labetalol
d. phenoxybenzamine
e. prazosin

*α 2*

*Irreversible Blockade X + I_NC*

**285.** The reversible cholinesterase inhibitor indicated in the treatment of Alzheimer's disease is

a.  tacrine
b.  edrophonium
c.  neostigmine
d.  pyridostigmine
e.  ambenonium

**286.** Hypotension, bradycardia, respiratory depression, and muscle weakness, all unresponsive to atropine and neostigmine, would most likely be due to

a.  diazoxide
b.  isofluorophate
c.  tubocurarine
d.  nicotine
e.  pilocarpine

**287.** Ritodrine hydrochloride is used in the treatment of

a.  Parkinson's disease
b.  bronchial asthma
c.  depression
d.  hypertension
e.  premature labor

**288.** The skeletal muscle relaxant that acts directly on the contractile mechanism of the muscle fibers is

a.  gallamine
b.  baclofen
c.  pancuronium
d.  cyclobenzaprine
e.  dantrolene

**289.** A predictably dangerous side effect of nadolol that constitutes a contraindication to its clinical use in susceptible patients is the induction of

a.  hypertension
b.  cardiac arrhythmia
c.  asthmatic attacks
d.  respiratory depression
e.  hypersensitivity

**290.** All the following drugs are used topically in the treatment of chronic wide-angle glaucoma. Which of these agents reduces intraocular pressure by decreasing the formation of the aqueous humor?

a.  betaxolol hydrochloride
b.  echothiophate iodide
c.  pilocarpine hydrochloride
d.  isofluorophate
e.  physostigmine salicylate

**291.** The cholinomimetic drug that is useful for treating postoperative abdominal distention and gastric atony is

a.  Ach
b.  methacholine
c.  carbachol
d.  bethanechol
e.  pilocarpine

**292.** Neostigmine will effectively antagonize skeletal muscle relaxation produced by

a.  metocurine
b.  succinylcholine
c.  diazepam
d.  baclofen
e.  nicotine

**293.** Pralidoxime chloride is a drug that

a.  reduces the vesicular stores of catecholamines in adrenergic and dopaminergic neurons
b.  blocks the active transport of choline into cholinergic neurons
c.  reactivates cholinesterases that have been inhibited by organophosphate cholinesterase inhibitors
d.  stimulates the activity of phospholipase C with increased formation of inositol triphosphate
e.  inhibits the reuptake of biogenic amines into nerve terminals

**294.** Which of the following antimuscarinic drugs is used by inhalation in the treatment of bronchial asthma?

a.  dicyclomine hydrochloride
b.  cyclopentolate hydrochloride
c.  ipratropium bromide
d.  methscopolamine bromide
e.  trihexyphenidyl hydrochloride

**295.** The cholinesterase inhibitor that is used in the diagnosis of myasthenia gravis is

a.  edrophonium chloride
b.  ambenonium chloride
c.  malathion
d.  physostigmine salicylate
e.  pyridostigmine bromide

**296.** Epinephrine may be mixed with certain anesthetics, such as procaine, in order to

a.  stimulate local wound repair
b.  promote hemostasis
c.  enhance their interaction with neural membranes and their ability to depress nerve conduction
d.  retard their systemic absorption
e.  facilitate their distribution along nerves and fascial planes

**297.** The skeletal muscles that are most sensitive to the action of tubocurarine are the

a.  muscles of the trunk
b.  muscles of the arms and legs
c.  respiratory muscles
d.  muscles of the head, neck, and face
e.  abdominal muscles

**298.** The drug of choice for the treatment of anaphylactic shock is

a.  epinephrine
b.  norepinephrine (NE)
c.  isoproterenol
d.  diphenhydramine
e.  atropine

**299.** Both phentolamine and prazosin

a. are competitive antagonists at $\alpha_1$-adrenergic receptors
b. have potent direct vasodilator actions on vascular smooth muscle
c. enhance gastric acid secretion through a histamine-like effect
d. cause hypotension and bradycardia
e. are used chronically for the treatment of primary hypertension

**300.** Pancuronium bromide may cause an increased heart rate due to

a. a reflex response to hypotension caused by the drug
b. blockade of nicotinic-neural ($N_N$) receptors in parasympathetic ganglia
c. its vagolytic action on the heart
d. a digitalis-like action on the myocardium
e. direct stimulation of the vasomotor center in the brainstem

**DIRECTIONS:** Each numbered question or incomplete statement below is NEGATIVELY phrased. Select the **one best** lettered response.

**301.** All the following are possible effects of low doses of nicotine (from smoking tobacco products) EXCEPT

a. increased tone and motor activity of the intestine
b. stimulation of respiratory rate and depth *(Banis)*
c. stimulation of catecholamine release from the adrenal medulla
d. bradycardia *(↑ ITR)*
e. nausea and vomiting

**302.** All the following drugs have significant antimuscarinic effects EXCEPT

a. diphenhydramine
b. pyridostigmine *(Cholinomedic)*
c. meperidine *(opioid)*
d. amitriptyline
e. thioridazine

**303.** All the following neuromuscular blocking agents are biotransformed by either deacetylation or ester hydrolysis, which results in the formation of an active skeletal muscle relaxant, EXCEPT *(Hoffmann ↓ zero order Kinetics)*

a. atracurium besylate
b. pancuronium bromide
c. pipecuronium bromide
d. succinylcholine chloride
e. vecuronium bromide

**304.** All the following statements are true concerning isoproterenol EXCEPT that

a. it is readily absorbed when administered parenterally or by aerosol
b. it lowers peripheral resistance and diastolic blood pressure
c. it relaxes bronchial smooth muscle
d. it is biotransformed primarily in the liver by MAO
e. it is used as a cardiac stimulant in heart block and cardiogenic shock after myocardial infarction (MI)

**305.** Propranolol is either contraindicated in, or should be used with caution in, all the following disease states EXCEPT

a. hypoglycemia
b. Raynaud's phenomenon
c. bronchial asthma
d. congestive heart failure (CHF)
e. angina pectoris *(↓ ITR ↓ BP ↓ Myocardial O₂ demand)*

**306.** All the following structures respond to β-adrenergic receptor stimulation EXCEPT

a. the ciliary muscle of the iris
b. the radial muscle of the iris
c. bronchial muscle
d. the atrioventricular (AV) node
e. the sinoatrial (SA) node

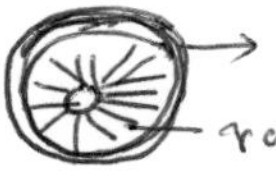

*radial fibres (α) constricts ↓ Mydriasis*

**307.** All the following drugs act within sympathetic neurons to depress neurotransmitter release and are used to treat hypertension EXCEPT

a. guanadrel
b. metyrosine
c. selegiline    *MAO I*
d. reserpine
e. guanethidine

**308.** Atropine and scopolamine will block all the effects of Ach listed below EXCEPT

a. bradycardia
b. salivary secretion
c. bronchoconstriction
d. skeletal muscle contraction
e. miosis

**309.** Propranolol is indicated for use in patients with all the following conditions EXCEPT

a. hypertension
b. angina pectoris
c. glaucoma
d. migraine headaches
e. supraventricular and ventricular arrhythmias

**310.** All the following statements are true concerning the use of therapeutic oral doses of amphetamine EXCEPT

a. the drug may cause hypotension by decreasing both systolic and diastolic blood pressure
b. wakefulness, alertness, headache, and agitation are common CNS effects of the drug
c. anorexia is a common effect of this drug
d. narcolepsy and attention deficit hyperactivity disorder (ADHD) are approved indications for amphetamine
e. amphetamine induces the release of biogenic amines from storage sites in neuron terminals

**311.** All the following statements are accurate characterizations of ephedrine EXCEPT that it

a. is used as a decongestant
b. can cause insomnia, restlessness, agitation, and tremors
c. can increase systemic blood pressure
d. is rapidly biotransformed by both COMT and MAO
e. will relax the smooth muscles of the bronchial tree

*Not
↓
Thats why they have central effects*

*gan blon blocker*

**312.** All the following are possible effects of mecamylamine EXCEPT

a. arteriolar vasodilatation
b. mydriasis and cycloplegia
c. constipation and urinary retention
d. tachycardia
e. skeletal muscle weakness

**313.** All the following statements are true concerning dobutamine hydrochloride EXCEPT that it

a. is a selective agonist at $\beta_1$-adrenergic receptors
b. activates dopaminergic receptors in renal and mesenteric vascular beds
c. is used to increase cardiac output in patients with severe cardiac failure
d. must be given by IV administration
e. may cause tachycardia and anginal pain

*Do some*

**314.** All the following are effects elicited by activation of the parasympathetic nervous system EXCEPT

a. decreased heart rate
b. increased tone of longitudinal smooth muscles of the intestine
c. contraction of skeletal muscles → NM / Ach ??
d. contraction of the detrusor of the urinary bladder
e. secretion of fluid from the lacrimal glands

**315.** All the following compounds are believed to function as cotransmitters or neuromodulators that exist with Ach or NE in neurons of the autonomic nervous system (ANS) EXCEPT

a. vasoactive intestinal peptide (VIP)
b. adenosine triphosphate (ATP)
c. neuropeptide Y (NPY)
d. substance P
e. serotonin (5-hydroxytryptamine [5-HT])

*Separate    Neurotransmitter*

**DIRECTIONS:** Each group of questions below consists of lettered headings followed by a set of numbered items. For each numbered item, select the **one** lettered heading with which it is **most** closely associated. Each lettered heading may be used **once, more than once, or not at all.**

### Questions 316–317

For each patient, which drug was given?

a. diazepam
b. doxazosin
c. scopolamine
d. cyclobenzaprine
e. propantheline
f. atracurium
g. atenolol
h. baclofen
i. timolol
j. phentolamine

**316.** A 65- year-old male complains of "losing" his vision. Retinal examination reveals optic nerve cupping. Peripheral vision loss is observed on visual field tests, and his intraocular pressure is increased. Following treatment with a drug, he has improved visual acuity and decreased intraocular pressure. *Timolol*

**317.** A 30-year-old female is being prepared for anesthesia before exploratory surgery for a mass in her neck. In addition to using an inhalation anesthetic, a drug is given that causes complete paralysis of the skeletal muscles.
*( Atracurion )*

### Questions 318–320

For each anatomic site listed, select the catecholamine neurotransmitter found in the highest amounts.

a. DM
b. 5-HT
c. epinephrine
d. NE
e. Ach

**318.** Adrenergic fibers    *NE*

**319.** Adrenal medulla    *EP*

**320.** Caudate nucleus    *Dopa*

## Questions 321–323

The figure below illustrates proposed sites of action of drugs. For each drug listed, select the site of action that the drug is most likely to inhibit (α = alpha receptor; β = beta receptor; COMT = catechol-O-methyltransferase; MAO = monoamine oxidase; NE = norepinephrine; NMN = normetanephrine).

*c* **321.** Reserpine

*e* **322.** Esmolol

*c* **323.** Tranylcypromine

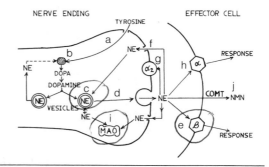

SYMPATHETIC NEUROEFFECTOR JUNCTION

## Questions 324–326

For each patient, select the mechanism of action most likely associated with the administered drug:

a. α-adrenergic antagonist
b. β-adrenergic antagonist
c. calcium (Ca) channel antagonist
d. carbonic anhydrase inhibitor
e. histamine₁ (H₁) receptor antagonist
f. H₂ receptor antagonist
g. MAOI
h. sodium/potassium (Na⁺/K⁺) adenosine triphosphatase (ATPase) inhibitor
i. Na⁺ channel antagonist
j. serotonin receptor antagonist

*e* **324.** A 16-year-old female has a two-year history of runny nose and itchy eyes from mid-August through mid-October. Chlorpheniramine is given and provides symptomatic relief.  *H₂ → Antagonist*

**325.** A 66-year-old male with a one-year history of essential hypertension has minimal response to diet and a diuretic. His blood pressure is now 160/105 mmHg. The diuretic is discontinued, and prazosin is given.  *α, Blocker* *Selective*

**326.** During the past year, a 38-year-old female has become progressively depressed and now refuses to leave her house. Physical examination and blood chemistries are negative. She is given tranylcypromine, which diminishes her depression and enables her to leave her house.  *MAOI*

## Questions 327–329

For each of the neurotransmitters below, select the amino acid from which it is synthesized.

a. tyrosine
b. serine
c. histidine
d. tryptophan
e. hydroxyproline

*a* **327.** Epinephrine  *Tyrosine*

*c* **328.** Histamine  *Histidine  c*

*d* **329.** Serotonin  *Tryptophan  b*

## Questions 330–332

Match the descriptions of use with the appropriate drug.

a. tropicamide
b. methylphenidate
c. propantheline
d. ritodrine
e. guanethidine

*e* **330.** Used as an antihypertensive drug  *Guanethidine*

**331.** Used in the treatment of gastrointestinal (GI) hypermotility  *propantheline*

**332.** Used as an adjunct in the therapy of hyperkinetic syndromes  (*Methylphenidate*)

## Questions 333–335

For each of the drugs below, select its appropriate site of action in the Ach system diagrammed.

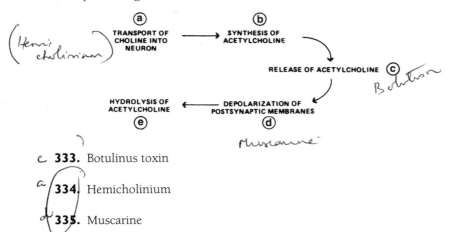

(*Hemicholinium*) ⓐ TRANSPORT OF CHOLINE INTO NEURON ⟶ ⓑ SYNTHESIS OF ACETYLCHOLINE ⟶ RELEASE OF ACETYLCHOLINE ⓒ *Botulism*

ⓔ HYDROLYSIS OF ACETYLCHOLINE ⟵ DEPOLARIZATION OF POSTSYNAPTIC MEMBRANES ⓓ  *Muscarine*

*c* **333.** Botulinus toxin

*a* **334.** Hemicholinium

*d* **335.** Muscarine

# Autonomic Nervous System

## Answers

**280. The answer is c.** (*DiPalma, 4/e, pp 102, 110, 116–119.*) Stimulation of both the contractile and rhythmic effects of epinephrine on the heart is mediated through activation of postsynaptic $\beta_1$-adrenergic receptors. These receptor sites mediate an epinephrine-induced increased firing rate of the SA node, increased conduction velocity through the AV node and the His-Purkinje system, and increased contractility and conduction velocity of atrial and ventricular muscle. Epinephrine activation of $\alpha$-adrenoceptors does not affect cardiac function. $\beta_2$-adrenergic receptors play a minor role in cardiac stimulation. They are more important in the relaxation of tracheobronchial smooth muscle, relaxation of the detrusor of the urinary bladder, dilation of arterioles that serve skeletal muscles, and increased secretion of insulin by the pancreas. Lipolysis in fat cells and melatonin secretion by the pineal gland appear to involve stimulation of $\beta_3$-adrenergic receptors.

**281. The answer is b.** (*AMA Drug Evaluations Annual, 1993, pp 2057, 2065. DiPalma, 4/e, pp 155, 160–161.*) Echothiophate iodide is a long-acting (irreversible) cholinesterase inhibitor. It is used topically in the eye for the treatment of various types of glaucoma. Maximum reduction of intraocular pressure occurs within 24 h and the effect may persist for several days. The drug is a water-soluble compound, which affords it a practical advantage over the lipid-soluble isoflurophate (another cholinesterase inhibitor used to treat glaucoma).

**282. The answer is e.** (*DiPalma, 4/e, p 168.*) All the drugs listed in the question are used as antiemetics. Chlorpromazine is a general antiemetic, used orally, rectally, or by injection for the control of nausea and vomiting that is caused by conditions that are not necessarily defined. Ondansetron is indicated in the oral or IV route for the prevention of nausea and vomiting caused by cancer chemotherapy. Diphenhydramine and dimenhydrinate are used orally for the active and prophylactic treatment of motion sickness.

Scopolamine is a transdermal preparation used in the prevention of motion sickness. The drug is incorporated into a bandagelike adhesive unit that is placed behind the ear. The scopolamine delivered in this manner is well absorbed and maintains an effect for up to 72 h. Other drugs that are prepared for transdermal delivery include clonidine (an antihypertensive agent), estradiol (an estrogen), fentanyl (an opioid analgesic), nicotine (a smoking deterrent), nitroglycerin (an antianginal drug), and testosterone (an androgen).

**283. The answer is e.** (*DiPalma, 4/e, pp 137–138.*) With the exception of acebutolol—which is classified as a "cardioselective," or selective, $\beta_1$-adrenergic blocking agent—all the listed drugs are considered to be nonselective $\beta$-adrenergic blocking agents because they will competitively antagonize agonists at both $\beta_1$- and $\beta_2$-adrenergic receptor sites. Labetalol is unique in that it is, at therapeutic doses, also a competitive antagonist at $\alpha_1$-adrenergic receptors. The drug has more potent blocking activity at $\beta$-adrenoceptors; the potency ratio for $\alpha:\beta$ blockade is 1:3 for the oral route and 1:7 after IV administration. Similar to the other $\beta$-adrenergic blocking drugs, labetalol is indicated for the treatment of essential hypertension; however, because of the $\alpha_1$-adrenergic blocking activity, blood pressure is often decreased more in the standing than in the supine position and symptoms of postural hypotension can occur.

**284. The answer is d.** (*DiPalma, 4/e, pp 24, 138–143.*) Competitive antagonists produce a parallel shift to the right in the dose-response curve of an agonist without a reduction in the maximal effect. This type of inhibition of agonist response is due to the reversible binding of the antagonist with the affected receptor site(s); this is exemplified in the curve shown for the agonist NE (X) plus an antagonist ($N_C$). Noncompetitive antagonists prevent an agonist from inducing any effect at a given receptor site and thus reduce the number of receptor sites that can be stimulated by an agonist. These compounds produce a nonparallel shift in the dose-response curve of the agonist and a diminution in the maximum response, as shown by the curve labeled X + $I_{NC}$.

Norepinephrine (NE) contracts vascular smooth muscle by binding to and activating $\alpha_1$-adrenergic receptors. Phentolamine, prazosin, terazosin, and labetalol all bind to $\alpha_1$-adrenergic receptors, but fail to activate them. Since the action of these compounds is reversible, these drugs act as competitive antagonists of NE at these receptor sites. Phenoxybenzamine is an alkylating agent that forms a stable covalent bond with both $\alpha_1$- and $\alpha_2$-adrenergic receptors. This long-lasting receptor blockade cannot be overcome by competition with an agonist. Therefore, in contrast to the other drugs listed, blockade with phenoxybenzamine is not reversible, is referred to as *nonequilibrium receptor blockade*, and in the presence of an $\alpha$-adrenergic receptor agonist such as NE will result in a dose-response curve exemplified by curve $X + I_{NC}$.

**285. The answer is a.** (*DiPalma, 4/e, pp 159–160. Katzung, 7/e, p 994.*) Patients with Alzheimer's disease present with progressive impairment of memory and cognitive functions such as a lack of attention, disturbed language function, and an inability to complete common tasks. Although the exact defect in the central nervous system (CNS) has not been elucidated, evidence suggests that a reduction in cholinergic nerve function is largely responsible for the symptoms.

Tacrine has been found to be somewhat effective in patients with mild-to-moderate symptoms of this disease for improvement of cognitive functions. The drug is primarily a reversible cholinesterase inhibitor that increases the concentration of functional Ach in the brain. However, the pharmacology of tacrine is complex; the drug also acts as a muscarinic receptor modulator in that it has partial agonistic activity as well as weak antagonistic activity on muscarinic receptors in the CNS. In addition, tacrine appears to enhance the release of Ach from cholinergic nerves and it may alter the concentrations of other neurotransmitters such as DM and NE.

Of all the reversible cholinesterase inhibitors, only tacrine and physostigmine cross the blood-brain barrier in sufficient amounts to make these compounds useful for disorders involving the CNS. Physostigmine has been tried as a therapy for Alzheimer's disease; however, it is more commonly used to antagonize the effects of toxic concentrations of drugs with antimuscarinic properties, including atropine, antihistamines, phenothiazines, and tricyclic antidepressants. Neostigmine, pyridostigmine, and ambenonium are used mainly in the treatment of myasthenia gravis; edrophonium is useful for the diagnosis of this muscular disease.

**286. The answer is d.** (*DiPalma, 4/e, pp 151–153. Hardman and Limbird, 9/e, pp 192–193.*) Nicotine is a depolarizing ganglionic blocking agent that initially stimulates and then blocks nicotinic-muscular ($N_M$) (skeletal muscle)

*Basic fact  Nicotine*
*Nicotinic receptor*

and nicotinic-neural ($N_N$) (parasympathetic ganglia) cholinergic receptors. Blockade of the sympathetic division of the ANS results in arteriolar vasodilation, bradycardia, and hypotension. Blockade at the neuromuscular junction leads to muscle weakness and respiratory depression caused by interference with the function of the diaphragm and intercostal muscles. Atropine, a muscarinic receptor blocker, would be an effective antagonist, as would neostigmine, a cholinesterase inhibitor. Pilocarpine and isoflurophate are cholinomimetics and can be antagonized by atropine; the effects of tubocurarine can be inhibited by neostigmine. Diazoxide, a vasodilator, would cause tachycardia, rather than bradycardia.

**287. The answer is e.** (*AMA Drug Evaluations Annual, 1993, pp 1161–1163.*) Ritodrine hydrochloride is a selective $\beta_2$-adrenergic agonist that relaxes uterine smooth muscle. It also has the other effects attributable to $\beta$-adrenergic receptor stimulants, such as bronchodilation, cardiac stimulation, enhanced renin secretion, and hyperglycemia. Of all the selective $\beta_2$-adrenergic receptor agonists available in the United States, ritodrine is the only one approved for use in premature labor, although terbutaline sulfate is being evaluated in clinical trials for this indication.

**288. The answer is e.** (*DiPalma, 4/e, p 180. Katzung, 7/e, pp 447–448.*) There are three major classes of skeletal muscle relaxants: peripherally acting, centrally acting, and direct-acting. The peripherally acting drugs include the nondepolarizing (e.g., tubocurarine, gallamine, pancuronium) and depolarizing (e.g., succinylcholine, decamethonium) neuromuscular blockers that antagonize Ach at the muscle endplate (i.e., at $N_M$ receptors). Centrally acting skeletal muscle relaxants (e.g., diazepam, cyclobenzaprine, baclofen) interfere with transmission along the monosynaptic and polysynaptic neural pathways in the spinal cord. Dantrolene, the only direct-acting skeletal muscle relaxant, affects the excitation-contraction coupling mechanism of skeletal muscle by depressing the release of ionic Ca from the sarcoplasmic reticulum to the myoplasma. The drug is also useful in the prevention and management of malignant hyperthermia induced by general anesthetics.

*Key Word*

**289. The answer is c.** (*DiPalma, 4/e, p 136. Hardman and Limbird, 9/e, pp 233–235.*) The chief danger of therapy with $\beta$-adrenergic blocking agents such as nadolol and propranolol is associated with the blockade itself. $\beta$-adrenergic blockade results in an increase in airway resistance that can be fatal in asthmatic patients. Hypersensitivity reactions such as rash, fever, and purpura are rare and necessitate discontinuation of therapy.

**290. The answer is a.** (*AMA Drug Evaluations Annual, 1993, pp 2057, 2059–2061, 2065. Hardman and Limbird, 9/e, pp 146–147, 167.*) When applied topically to the eye, both the direct-acting cholinomimetic agents (e.g., pilocarpine) and those cholinomimetic drugs that act by inhibition of AchE (e.g., echothiophate, isoflurophate, and physostigmine) cause miosis by contracting the sphincter muscle of the iris and reduction of ocular pressure by contraction of the ciliary muscle. In patients with glaucoma, this latter effect permits greater drainage of the aqueous humor through the trabecular meshwork in the canal of Schlemm and a reduction in resistance to outflow of the aqueous humor. Certain β-adrenergic blocking agents (e.g., betaxolol, timolol, and levobunolol) applied to the eye are also very useful in treating chronic wide-angle glaucoma. These drugs appear to act by decreasing the secretion (or formation) of the aqueous humor by antagonizing the effect of circulating catecholamines on β-adrenergic receptors in the ciliary epithelium.

**291. The answer is d.** (*DiPalma, 4/e, pp 149–151. Hardman and Limbird, 9/e, pp 143–145.*) Of the four choline esters (Ach, methacholine, carbachol, and bethanechol), the latter two drugs have the greatest agonistic activity on muscarinic receptors of the GI tract and urinary bladder. Bethanechol is used orally or by subcutaneous injection as a stimulant of the smooth muscles of the GI tract (for cases of postoperative abdominal distention, gastric atony and retention or gastroparesis) and the urinary bladder (for nonobstructive postoperative and postpartum urinary retention). Carbachol is not used for these purposes due to significant activity at nicotinic receptors at autonomic ganglia; the drug is useful as a miotic for treating glaucoma and in certain types of ocular surgery. Acetycholine is occasionally used topically during cataract surgery; metacholine is used by inhalation for the diagnosis of bronchial hyperreactivity in patients who do not have clinically apparent asthma. Pilocarpine (a naturally occurring alkaloid) is a drug of choice for the treatment of glaucoma.

**292. The answer is a.** (*DiPalma, 4/e, pp 156–158. Hardman and Limbird, 9/e, pp 162–165.*) Anticholinesterase agents, such as neostigmine, will delay the catabolism of Ach released from parasympathetic autonomic and somatic nerve terminals. At the neuromuscular junction this results in increased competition for the $N_M$ receptors by Ach (the agonist) and the curariform drugs (the antagonists) such as tubocurarine, metocurine, and pancuronium. In addition, neostigmine has a direct stimulating action on the skeletal muscle junction, which enhances its ability to antagonize the competitive neuromuscular blockers. The activity of succinylcholine at the neuromuscular junction will be exacerbated by neostigmine, since succinylcholine is inactivated by AchE. The skeletal muscle relaxation that may result from toxic doses of nicotine-blocking $N_M$ receptors will be unaffected by neostigmine. Diazepam and baclofen are centrally acting skeletal muscle relaxants whose effects are not altered by the peripheral actions of neostigmine.

**293. The answer is c.** (*DiPalma, 4/e, pp 160–162. Hardman and Limbird, 9/e, pp 170–171.*) Organophosphate cholinesterase inhibitors react with both AchE and serum cholinesterase (pseudocholinesterase) by phosphorylating the enzymes, thus rendering them inactive, inasmuch as the phosphorylated enzyme hydrolyzes esters very slowly. Pralidoxime chloride (2-PAM Cl⁻) is an oxime derivative that can cause dephosphorylation of the enzyme if it is administered within a short time after the organophosphate. If not administered promptly, the phosphorylated enzyme will lose an alkyl or alkoxy group (a process called "aging"), leaving a more stable phosphorylated enzyme that then cannot be dephosphorylated. The time period during which this occurs depends upon the nature of the phosphoryl group and the rapidity with which the organophosphate compound affects the enzyme. This can be from a few seconds to several hours.

**294. The answer is c.** (*Hardman and Limbird, 9/e, pp 156–158.*) A wide variety of clinical conditions are treated with antimuscarinic drugs. Dicyclomine hydrochloride and methscopolamine bromide are used to reduce GI motility, although side effects—dryness of the mouth, loss of visual accommodation, and difficulty in urination—may limit their acceptance by patients. Cyclopentolate hydrochloride is used in ophthalmology for its mydriatic and cycloplegic properties during refraction of the eye. Trihexyphenidyl hydrochloride is one of the important antimuscarinic compounds used in the treatment of parkinsonism. For bronchodilation in patients with bronchial asthma and other bronchospastic diseases, ipratropium bromide is used by inhalation. Systemic adverse reactions are low since the actions are largely confined to the mouth and airways.

(Atropine Substitutes)

**295. The answer is a.** (*AMA Drug Evaluations Annual, 1993, pp 394–398.*) Although all the listed compounds inhibit the activity of the cholinesterases, only edrophonium chloride is used in the diagnosis of myasthenia gravis. The drug has a more rapid onset of action (1 to 3 min following IV administration) and a shorter duration of action (approximately 5 to 10 min) than pyridostigmine bromide and ambenonium chloride. It is more water-soluble than physostigmine salicylate and, therefore, produces no clinically significant adverse effects on the CNS. Pyridostigmine bromide and ambenonium chloride are used in the treatment of this muscle weakness disease. Physostigmine salicylate is indicated topically for the treatment of glaucomas and is also a valuable drug for treating toxicity of anticholinergic drugs such as atropine. Malathion is an anticholinesterase that is used topically for the treatment of head lice and is never used internally.

**296. The answer is d.** (*DiPalma, 4/e, pp 368, 371.*) The addition of a vasoconstrictor, such as epinephrine or phenylephrine, to certain short-acting, local anesthetics is a common practice in order to prevent the rapid systemic absorption of the local anesthetic, to prolong the local action, and to decrease the potential systemic reactions. Some local anesthetics cause vasodilation, which allows more compound to escape the tissue and enter the blood. Procaine (Novocaine) is an ester-type local anesthetic with a short duration of action due to rather rapid biotransformation in the plasma by cholinesterases. The duration of action of the drug during infiltration anesthesia is greatly increased by the addition of epinephrine, which reduces the vasodilation caused by procaine.

**297. The answer is d.** (*DiPalma, 4/e, p 176. Hardman and Limbird, 9/e, pp 183–185.*) Flaccid paralysis of all skeletal muscles can be produced by the IV administration of large doses of a neuromuscular blocking agent such as tubocurarine. However, not all skeletal musculature is equally sensitive to the action of these drugs. The muscles that produce fine movements—e.g., the extraocular muscles, fingers, and muscles of the head, face, and neck—are most sensitive to these drugs. Muscles of the trunk, abdomen, and extremities are relaxed next, and the respiratory muscles (i.e., the intercostals and the diaphragm) are the most resistant to the action of tubocurarine.

**298. The answer is a.** (*AMA Drug Evaluations Annual, 1993, pp 1834–1835.*) Epinephrine is the drug of choice to relieve the symptoms of an acute, systemic, immediate hypersensitivity reaction to an allergen (anaphylactic shock). Subcutaneous administration of a 1:1000 solution of epinephrine rapidly relieves itching and urticaria and may save the life of the patient when laryngeal edema and bronchospasm threaten suffocation and severe hypotension and cardiac arrhythmias become life-endangering. NE, isoproterenol, and atropine are ineffective therapies. Angioedema is responsive to antihistamines (e.g., diphenhydramine), but epinephrine is necessary in the event of a severe reaction.

**299.  The answer is a.** (*AMA Drug Evaluations Annual, 1993, pp 576–578. DiPalma, 4/e, pp 139–140, 143, 475–476.*) Phentolamine is a nonselective α-adrenergic receptor blocker (i.e., it has affinity for both $\alpha_1$- and $\alpha_2$-adrenergic receptor sites). It also has a prominent direct relaxant (musculotropic spasmolytic) effect on arterioles, which results in vasodilation and reflex tachycardia. In addition, phentolamine can block the effects of serotonin and will increase hydrochloric acid and pepsin secretion from the stomach. Phentolamine is used for the short-term control of hypertension in patients with pheochromocytoma (i.e., a type of secondary hypertension); because of the high incidence of tachycardia associated with the compound, it is not used chronically for the treatment of primary hypertension. Prazosin is a selective $\alpha_1$-adrenergic receptor antagonist that, at therapeutic doses, has little activity at $\alpha_2$-adrenergic receptors and clinically insignificant direct vasodilating activity. The drug does not cause the other effects attributed to phentolamine. Most importantly, it produces less tachycardia than does phentolamine and, therefore, is useful in the treatment of primary hypertension.

**300.  The answer is c.** (*DiPalma, 4/e, p 177.*) Unlike most other neuromuscular blocking agents, cardioacceleration may be observed with both pancuronium bromide and gallamine triethiodide). The increased heart rate that may be observed with pancuronium appears to be primarily due to an atropine-like antimuscarinic (vagolytic) action on the heart, although other mechanisms have been proposed including (1) release of catecholamines from postganglionic adrenergic cardiac fibers, (2) blockade of neuronal norepinephrine reuptake, and (3) a mild ganglionic ($N_N$) stimulant effect. Pancuronium does not cause hypotension, has little ganglionic blocking activity, does not affect the myocardium like digitalis, and does not cross the blood-brain barrier in order to stimulate the vasomotor center.

**301. The answer is d.** (*DiPalma, 4/e, pp 151–153. Hardman and Limbird, 9/e, pp 192–193.*) Nicotine is a depolarizing ganglionic blocking agent; that is, it stimulates $N_N$ receptors in low doses and predominantly blocks at high dose levels. The effect of nicotine on a particular tissue or organ depends on the relative contribution to function made by each division of the ANS. The effects on the cardiovascular system are complex. Stimulation of the cardiac vagal ganglia causes bradycardia. This is countered by sympathetic stimulation to the heart (tachycardia), blood vessels (vasoconstriction), and adrenal medulla (catecholamine release: tachycardia and vasoconstriction). Thus the net effect of nicotine on the heart is tachycardia, not bradycardia. Low doses of nicotine augment respiration by excitation of the chemoreceptors of the carotid body and aortic arch. Higher doses also stimulate the medullary respiratory center and increase respiration through CNS activity. Large amounts of nicotine cause respiratory failure from medullary paralysis and blockade of the skeletal muscles of respiration.

**302. The answer is b.** (*DiPalma, 4/e, pp 158, 194, 277, 278, 292, 293.*) Many compounds from diverse pharmacologic categories elicit antimuscarinic (anticholinergic) effects. As an example, diphenhydramine (an antihistamine), meperidine (an opioid analgesic), amitriptyline (an antidepressant), and thioridazine (an antipsychotic) all produce clinically significant antimuscarinic effects. In some cases, these become annoying adverse reactions, e.g., dryness of the mouth and tachycardia, as seen with amitriptyline. In other instances this property can be useful (e.g., reduced nasal secretions enhance the utility of diphenhydramine in cold and allergy treatments).

Pyridostigmine does not have antimuscarinic activity; rather, it *produces* muscarinic and nicotinic effects. This drug is an indirect-acting cholinomimetic agent that inhibits the activity of AchE and plasma cholinesterase, the enzymes that hydrolyze Ach. Pyridostigmine is used as the drug of choice for oral therapy of myasthenia gravis.

**303. The answer is a.** (*DiPalma, 4/e, pp 177–179.*) Many of the older neuromuscular blocking agents, such as tubocurarine chloride, metocurine iodide, and gallamine triethiodide are very stable in the body and therefore are not biotransformed to a significant extent; these drugs are eliminated unchanged from the body primarily by the kidney. Doxacurium chloride is a newer neuromuscular blocking agent that is not biotransformed; its routes of elimination are through the bile and urine. Most of the other neuromuscular blocking drugs are biotransformed by either deacetylation or by hydrolysis of ester groups. Pancuronium, pipecuronium, and vecuronium are partially deacetylated to the active products 3-hydroxy pancuronium, 3-desacetyl pipecuronium, and 3-desacetyl vecuronium, respectively. Succinylcholine is hydrolyzed by cholinesterases to form succinylmonocholine, an active skeletal muscle relaxant. Atracurium and mivacurium chloride are metabolized by ester hydrolysis to inactive products.

**304. The answer is d.** (*DiPalma, 4/e, pp 114–119, 121–122. Hardman and Limbird, 9/e, pp 212–213.*) Isoproterenol is a nonselective β-adrenergic receptor agonist. Cardiac stimulation (through $\beta_1$-receptors), relaxed bronchial smooth muscle, and vasodilation (through $\beta_2$-receptors) are typical effects observed following the administration of the drug. Based on these effects, isoproterenol is used as a cardiac stimulant in heart block and shock (by injection) and as a bronchodilator in respiratory disorders (by inhalation). The drug is short-acting since it is metabolized primarily and efficiently by COMT. It is a relatively poor substrate for MAO, however.

**305. The answer is e.** (*DiPalma, 4/e, p 136. Hardman and Limbird, 9/e, pp 235–237.*) Propranolol is a competitive antagonist of both $\beta_1$- and $\beta_2$-adrenergic receptors. Since the sympathetic division of the ANS may be a vital component in support of cardiac performance in many patients with CHF, $\beta_1$-adrenergic blockade may precipitate more severe depression of cardiac function. The $\beta_2$-adrenoceptors in the bronchioles of patients with bronchospastic disease (e.g., bronchial asthma, chronic bronchitis, emphysema) are important in mediating bronchodilation; thus, blockade of these receptors may cause a severe increase in airway resistance, thereby decreasing pulmonary function in such patients, which may be life-threatening. Propranolol should also be used with caution in diabetic patients who are prone to hypoglycemia since β-adrenergic blockers may mask the warning signs of acute hypoglycemia (e.g., tachycardia). Some patients who use propranolol and other β-adrenergic blockers complain of cold extremities. Because these drugs may mildly elevate peripheral resistance, they should be used with caution in patients with vasospastic diseases such as Raynaud's phenomenon and acrocyanosis. There is no contraindication or warning concerning the use of propranolol in angina pectoris; rather, propranolol and other β-adrenergic blocking agents are indicated for the treatment of this disease. There have been reports, however, of exacerbation of angina following abrupt discontinuation of these drugs.

**306.** **The answer is b.** (*DiPalma, 4/e, pp 102–103.*) The radial muscle of the iris contains predominantly α-adrenergic receptors; when exposed to such α-receptor agonists as phenylephrine, the muscle contracts, resulting in mydriasis. Miosis occurs when the ciliary muscle, which contains β-receptors, relaxes. Bronchial muscle, the AV node, and the SA node are among other sites that contain β-receptors and respond to β-adrenergic agonists.

**307.** **The answer is c.** (*DiPalma, 4/e, pp 131, 143–145, 318. Hardman and Limbird, 9/e, p 512.*) Selegiline (also known as *deprenyl*) is a selective MAOI that is used to treat Parkinson's disease. At recommended doses, the drug inhibits MAO type B (found mainly in the brain), with little effect on MAO type A (found predominantly in the intestine and liver). Inhibition of MAO will tend to raise the pool of catecholamine neurotransmitters (NE, DM) available for release by sympathetic neurons.

Guanadrel and guanethidine are adrenergic neuronal blocking drugs that deplete stores of neurotransmitters in sympathetic neurons by competing with catecholamine for binding sites within the storage vesicles. When the sympathetic neurons are depolarized, less neurotransmitter is available to be released. Both of these compounds are used to treat essential hypertension.

Reserpine causes depletion of NE and DM by binding to the membrane of the storage vesicles and irreversibly inhibiting the magnesium-dependent ATP transport process that is responsible for catecholamine uptake into the neuronal vesicles. Like guanethidine and guanadrel, reserpine is indicated for the treatment of essential hypertension.

Metyrosine is a competitive antagonist of tyrosine hydroxylase, the enzyme that converts tyrosine to 3,4-dihydroxyphenylalanine (dopa), and the rate-limiting step in the formation of NE and epinephrine. Metyrosine is used to treat patients with pheochromocytoma, a tumor of the adrenal medulla that produces excessive quantities of these catecholamines and results in hypertension. This compound is not recommended for use in essential hypertension or in hypertension secondary to diseases other than functional adrenal tumors.

**308.** **The answer is d.** (*DiPalma, 4/e, pp 164–166. Hardman and Limbird, 9/e, pp 142–143.*) Ach will stimulate both muscarinic and nicotinic receptors. Skeletal muscle contraction is mediated through nicotinic-muscular ($N_M$) receptors, and ganglionic stimulation is an effect of nicotinic-neural

($N_N$) receptors. All the other effects listed in the question occur following muscarinic receptor activation and will be blocked by atropine and scopolamine, both of which are muscarinic receptor antagonists. Skeletal muscle contraction will not be affected by these drugs; rather, a neuromuscular blocker (e.g., tubocurarine) is required to antagonize this effect of Ach.

**309. The answer is c.** *(DiPalma, 4/e, p 138. Hardman and Limbird, 9/e, pp 236–237.)* In addition to its usefulness in the treatment of hypertension, angina pectoris, supraventricular and ventricular arrhythmias, and in the prophylaxis of migraine headaches, propranolol is indicated for use in hypertrophic subaortic stenosis and pheochromocytoma and to reduce cardiovascular mortality following a MI. Propranolol is the β-adrenergic blocker with the greatest *membrane stabilizing* activity (also known as *local anesthetic activity*). Propranolol applied topically to membranes, such as the cornea, would anesthetize the area; in the case of the eye, this would be detrimental to the patient. Therefore, this drug is not used for the treatment of glaucoma. Other β-adrenergic blockers that do not have membrane stabilizing activity—including timolol, betaxolol, and levobunolol—are useful for this purpose. All of these are administered as drops to the eye.

**310. The answer is a.** *(DiPalma, 4/e, pp 127, 268–269. Hardman and Limbird, 9/e, pp 219–221.)* Amphetamine and its derivative methamphetamine are sympathomimetic compounds that promote the release of various biogenic amines (e.g., DM, NE, 5-HT) from storage vesicles in neurons and are agonists at α- and β-adrenergic receptor sites. Oral administration of amphetamine *raises* both systolic and diastolic blood pressure and may cause heart rate to slow reflexly. The drug is a potent CNS stimulant and evokes excitation, increased alertness, elevation of mood, and insomnia. Anorexia (a loss of appetite) is a common manifestation of amphetamine use and the drug is widely used in the treatment of obesity, although such use is questionable owing to the high potential for abuse of the compound. Amphetamine is approved for use in narcolepsy, a disease characterized by sudden attacks of sleep, and in ADHD, a syndrome in children characterized by impulsive behavior, short attention span, and excessive motor activity.

**311. The answer is d.** *(DiPalma, 4/e, pp 126–127. Hardman and Limbird, 9/e, p 221.)* Ephedrine directly stimulates both α- and β-adrenergic receptors and causes release of NE from adrenergic neurons. Qualitatively its pharmacologic effects resemble those of epinephrine; the drug can increase blood pressure by both vasoconstriction and cardiac stimulation and it will relax bronchiolar smooth muscle. Ephedrine is less potent than epinephrine and the effects observed are usually slower in onset and of longer duration than those of epinephrine. Also in contrast to epinephrine, ephedrine is used orally in many cough and cold preparations for its decongestant activity.

*ephedrine*

?

Ephedrine is quite lipid-soluble compared with epinephrine and will pass through the blood-brain barrier and may cause stimulation of the CNS. Because epinephrine lacks a catechol moiety, it is not biotransformed by COMT and the methyl substitution on the α carbon allows the drug to resist oxidation by MAO.

**312. The answer is e.** (*DiPalma, 4/e, pp 170–172.*) Mecamylamine is a competitive antagonist of Ach at ganglionic cholinergic receptors ($N_N$) and will reduce the activity of both the parasympathetic and the sympathetic divisions of the ANS. Because the sympathetic nervous system controls vascular reactivity, mecamylamine will block sympathetic tone to the arterioles, resulting in vasodilation and decreased blood pressure; because of this effect, the drug is used (although rarely today) for the treatment of chronic hypertension. Parasympathetic tone predominates at most other effector structures and, therefore, this drug will affect the heart (tachycardia), eye (mydriasis and cycloplegia), GI tract (constipation), urinary bladder (retention of urine), salivary glands (xerostomia), and sweat glands (anhidrosis); these are all adverse manifestations of the compound. Since the nerve pathway to skeletal muscle involves only a single cholinergic motor nerve and no ganglia, and since mecamylamine does not compete with Ach for binding to $N_M$ receptors at the myoneural junction, mecamylamine will have no effect on skeletal muscle tone.

*key*

*Wow*

**313. The answer is b.** (*AMA Drug Evaluations Annual, 1993, pp 672–673. DiPalma, 4/e, pp 122–123.*) At low therapeutic doses, this catecholamine is a selective agonist of myocardial ($\beta_1$-adrenergic) receptors; in higher doses, it will lose selectivity and stimulate $\beta_2$- and α-adrenergic receptor sites.

*tot* → ( Not dopaminergic receptors )

Although it is a structural derivative of DM, dobutamine has no activity on peripheral dopaminergic receptors.

The drug is not effective orally since it is rapidly biotransformed (plasma $t_{1/2}$ is approximately 2 min) by COMT and, therefore, must be given by IV infusion. It is used to improve myocardial function in patients with severe cardiac failure that has not responded to other treatment modalities. Cardiac adverse effects (e.g., tachycardia and anginal pain) may be observed and represent extensions of the pharmacologic activity of the drug.

**314. The answer is c.** (*Hardman and Limbird, 9/e, pp 115–117.*) Cholinergic impulses arising from the parasympathetic division of the ANS affect many tissues and organs throughout the body. Physiologically, this system is concerned primarily with the functions of energy conservation and maintenance of organ function during periods of reduced activity. Slowed heart rate, reduced blood pressure, increased GI motility, emptying of the urinary bladder, and stimulation of secretions from the pancreas, salivary glands, lacrimal glands, and bronchial and nasopharyngeal glands are all effects observed due to activation of this nervous system. However, skeletal muscle contraction is mediated through activation of the somatic nervous system, not the ANS.

Basic Point

**315. The answer is e.** (*Hardman and Limbird, 9/e, pp 134–137.*) Although Ach and NE are still considered the major neurotransmitters in the parasympathetic and sympathetic divisions of the ANS, respectively, other compounds that exist within autonomic nerve terminals have been found to be released simultaneously during nerve stimulation and are now viewed as cotransmitters or neuromodulators. For example, VIP is localized in a number of parasympathetic neurons, e.g., those that innervate sweat glands and salivary glands, and it appears to function as a cotransmitter with Ach in these structures. ATP and Ach both exist in cholinergic vesicles, and ATP is found within the granules of adrenergic fibers and in the adrenal medulla;

Basics

this compound is believed to be a neurotransmitter in the GI and genitourinary tracts. NPY appears associated with catecholamine-containing neurons and may contribute to vasoconstriction produced by stimulation of the sympathetic nervous system. Although less is known about the function of substance P, this small peptide is found within cholinergic nerves, especially at ganglionic sites, and may function as a neuromodulator. Serotonin is a neurotransmitter in the CNS; although it may play a role in regulating GI motility via peripheral serotonergic neurons, it has not been designated as a cotransmitter or neuromodulator in the ANS.

**316. The answer is i.** (_Hardman and Limbird, 9/e, p 237._) Timolol is a β-adrenergic receptor antagonist that does not show selectivity for $\beta_1$- or $\beta_2$-adrenoceptors; therefore, it decreases heart rate by blocking the action of endogenous catecholamines. Timolol, used to lower intraocular pressure in patients with chronic open-angle glaucoma (presumably by decreasing the production of aqueous humor), is more effective than many other types of drugs for this use.

**317. The answer is f.** (_Hardman and Limbird, 9/e, p 180._) Atracurium is a nondepolarizing neuromuscular blocking agent. Similar to tubocurarine, atracurium is a competitive antagonist of Ach at the $N_M$ receptors at the myoneural junction of skeletal muscle. At therapeutic doses, these drugs can induce complete paralysis of skeletal muscles, unlike the weaker, centrally acting skeletal muscle relaxants (e.g., diazepam, baclofen, cyclobenzaprine), which reduce spasms but do not completely block contractions. The primary therapeutic use of atracurium and other curariform drugs is as an adjunct in surgical anesthesia to relax the skeletal musculature and facilitate surgical manipulation.

**318–320. The answers are 318-d, 319-c, 320-a.** (_Hardman and Limbird, 9/e, pp 120–122._) DM is formed from tyrosine by hydroxylation with tyrosine hydroxylase and the removal of a $CO_2$ group by aromatic amino acid decarboxylase. The catecholamine is found in high concentrations in parts of the brain: the caudate nucleus, the median eminence, the tuberculum olfactorium, and the nucleus accumbens. DM appears to act as an inhibitory neurotransmitter.

NE is synthesized from DM by DM-β-oxidase, which hydroxylates the β-carbon. This enzyme is localized in the amine storage granules. NE is found in adrenergic fibers, the adrenal medulla, and in neurons in the locus ceruleus and lateral ventral tegmental fields of the CNS.

Epinephrine is synthesized from NE in the adrenal medulla. NE is methylated by phenylethanolamine-$N$-methyltransferase. Neurons containing this enzyme are also found in the CNS.

**321–323. The answers are 321-c, 322-e, 323-i.** (*DiPalma, 4/e, pp 130–133, 143–144, 299–300. Hardman and Limbird, 9/e, pp 238–239, 791.*) Reserpine is an adrenergic neuronal blocking agent that causes depletion of central and peripheral stores of NE and DM. Reserpine acts by irreversibly inhibiting the magnesium-dependent ATP transport process that functions as a carrier for biogenic amines from the cytoplasm of the neuron into the storage vesicle. Depletion of stored NE results in decreased sympathetic tone; therefore, reserpine causes vasodilation, bradycardia, and hypotension.

Esmolol hydrochloride is a competitive β-adrenergic receptor antagonist; it is selective for $\beta_1$-adrenoceptors. In contrast to pindolol, esmolol has little intrinsic sympathomimetic activity, and it differs from propranolol in that it lacks membrane stabilizing activity. Of all the β-adrenergic blocking drugs, this compound has the shortest duration of action; since it is an ester, it is hydrolyzed rapidly by plasma esterases and must be used by the IV route. Esmolol is approved only for the treatment of supraventricular arrhythmias.

Tranylcypromine sulfate is an antidepressant drug and an inhibitor of MAO. Its antidepressant effect is probably due to the accumulation of NE in the brain as a consequence of inhibition of the enzyme. The other MAOI currently used as an antidepressant is phenelzine sulfate.

**324. The answer is e.** (*Hardman and Limbird, 9/e, p 587. Katzung, 7/e, p 267.*) Chlorpheniramine is a competitive $H_1$ receptor antagonist that inhibits most responses of smooth muscle to histamine. $H_1$ receptor antagonists have negligible effects on $H_2$ or $H_3$ receptors.

**325. The answer is a.** (*Hardman and Limbird, 9/e, p 229. Katzung, 7/e, pp 165–166.*) Prazosin blocks $\alpha_1$-adrenergic receptors in arterioles and veins, causing a drop in peripheral vascular resistance and a decrease in venous return.

**326. The answer is g.** (*Hardman and Limbird, 9/e, pp 439–440.*) Most MAOIs are nonselective for MAO A and B. MAOIs mainly act on tissues regulated by sympathomimetic amines and serotonin.

**327–329. The answers are 327-a, 328-c, 329-d.** (_DiPalma, 4/e, pp 107, 186, 200. Hardman and Limbird, 9/e, pp 120 , 250, 582–583._) Epinephrine is made from tyrosine in a series of steps through dopa, DM, NE, and finally epinephrine. The conversion of tyrosine to dopa by tyrosine hydroxylase is the rate-limiting step in this pathway. Epinephrine constitutes about 80% of the catecholamines in the adrenal medulla. The enzyme that synthesizes epinephrine from NE is also found in certain areas of the CNS.

Histamine, formed by the decarboxylation of histidine, is stored in mast cells and basophils; some other tissues can synthesize histamine but do not store it. Histamine is released from sensitized mast cells during allergic reactions.

Serotonin is synthesized from tryptophan in two steps. Tryptophan is hydroxylated by tryptophan hydroxylase, and 5-hydroxytryptophan is decarboxylated to give serotonin. Most serotonin in the body is found in the enterochromaffin cells of the intestinal tract and the pineal gland. Platelets take up and store serotonin but do not synthesize it.

**330–332. The answers are 330-e, 331-c, 332-b.** (_DiPalma, 4/e, pp 128, 144–145, 168–169. Hardman and Limbird, 9/e, pp 156, 221, 790._) Guanethidine inhibits the activity of peripheral sympathetic nerves by impairing neurotransmitter (norepinephrine) release. Chronic administration causes depletion of NE from intraneuronal storage granules by displacement. Reduced activity of the sympathetic division of the ANS leads to bradycardia, vasodilation, and reduced systemic blood pressure.

Propantheline is a semisynthetic antimuscarinic agent, similar to atropine and scopolamine. Its major use is in the treatment of peptic ulcer and GI hypermotility. Although less potent than atropine for this purpose, it will produce adverse effects commonly associated with the antimuscarinic group (e.g., xerostomia, tachycardia, and dilated pupils).

Methylphenidate is structurally and pharmacologically related to amphetamine. It is used in both children and adults who are characterized as having attention deficit disorder (ADD). It has been found to be effective in improving behavior, concentration, and learning ability in 70 to 80 % of children with ADD. Like amphetamine, it is a CNS stimulant and has significant potential for abuse.

**333–335. The answers are 333-c, 334-a, 335-d.** (_DiPalma, 4/e, pp 104–106, 150–151._) Ach is synthesized from acetyl-CoA and choline. Choline is taken up into the neurons by an active transport system. Hemicholinium blocks this uptake, depleting cellular choline, so that synthesis of Ach no longer occurs. Botulinus toxin comes from *Clostridium botulinum*, an organism that causes food poisoning. Botulinus toxin prevents the release of Ach from nerve endings by mechanisms that are not clear. Death occurs from respiratory failure caused by the inability of diaphragm muscles to contract.

Muscarine, an alkaloid from certain species of mushrooms, is a muscarinic receptor agonist. The compound has toxicologic importance; muscarine poisoning will produce all the effects associated with an overdose of Ach, e.g., bronchoconstriction, bradycardia, hypotension, excessive salivary and respiratory secretion, and sweating. Poisoning by muscarine is treated with atropine.

# LOCAL CONTROL SUBSTANCES

*(Autocoids NABAD. PG)* [handwritten]

**Note: In the classification of drugs, prototype drugs are marked with an asterisk (*).**

General Considerations
Concept of Autacoids
Histamine*
  Synthesis, distribution
  Localization, binding
  Release
  Inhibition of release → *rco* [handwritten]
  Receptors $H_1$, $H_2$, $H_3$
$H_1$-Receptor Antagonists
  Ethylenediamines
    Pyrilamine
    Tripelennamine*
  Aminoalkyl ethers
    Diphenhydramine*
    Dimenhydrinate
    Clemastine
  Alkylamines
    Chlorpheniramine*
    Dexchlorpheniramine
    Brompheniramine
    Triprolidine
  Piperazines
    Meclizine
    Cyclizine
    Hydroxyzine*
  Phenothiazines
    Promethazine*
    Trimeprazine
  Newer derivatives

Cyproheptadine*
Terfenadine*
Astemizole
Loratadine
Serotonin (5-hydroxytryptamine [5-HT])*
  Synthesis, storage, and metabolism
  Receptors
  5-HT agonists
    Sumatriptan → *rcd* *R migraine* [handwritten]
  5-HT antagonists
    Cyproheptadine → *rco* [handwritten]
    Methysergide
    Ondansetron
Ergot Alkaloids
  Source, chemistry
  Mechanism of action
  Adverse effects
  Dihydroergotamine
  Ergonovine
  Methylergonovine
Prostaglandins and Related Eicosanoids
  Chemistry, biosynthesis
  Biologic role
  Thromboxanes
  Leukotrienes
  Inhibitors of Eicosanoid Biosynthesis

Corticosteroids
Nonsteroidal anti-inflammatory
 drugs (NSAIDs)
Salicylates
 Aspirin
 Diflunisal
 Magnesium salicylate
 Salsalate
Propionic acids
 Fenoprofen
 Ibuprofen
 Ketoprofen
 Naproxen
Oxaprozin
Acetic acids
 Indomethacin
 Sulindac
 Tolmetin
 Diclofenac
Oxicams
 Piroxicam
Pyrazolone
 Phenylbutazone
Fenamates
 Meclofenamate
 Mefenamic acid

# Questions

**DIRECTIONS:** Each question below contains several suggested responses. Select the **one best** response to each question.

**336.** Sumatriptan succinate is effective for the treatment of acute migraine headaches by acting as

a. an antagonist at $\beta_1$- and $\beta_2$-adrenergic receptors
b. a selective antagonist at $H_1$ receptors
c. an inhibitor of prostacyclin synthase
d. an agonist at nicotinic receptors
e. a selective agonist at 5-HT$_{1D}$ receptors

**337.** Currently, three subtypes of histamine receptors are proposed: $H_1$ and $H_2$ receptors are found in peripheral tissues and the central nervous system (CNS), and $H_3$ receptors are found in the CNS. The second messenger pathway that mediates $H_1$ receptor stimulation is

a. increased formation of inositol trisphosphate
b. elevation of intracellular cyclic adenosine monophosphate (cAMP, cyclic AMP–adenosine 3′,5′-cyclic monophosphate)
c. activation of tyrosine kinases
d. inhibition of adenylate cyclase activity
e. activation of sodium ion flow into the cell

**338.** The pharmacologic effects of acetylsalicylic acid include

Basic fact

a. a reduction in elevated body temperature
b. promotion of platelet aggregation
c. alleviation of pain by stimulation of prostaglandin synthesis
d. efficacy equal to that of acetaminophen as an anti-inflammatory agent
e. less gastric irritation than other salicylates

**339.** Cyproheptadine is an antagonist at

a. dopamine ($D_1$) receptors
b. nicotine ($N_N$) receptors
c. benzodiazepine (BZ) receptors
d. histamine ($H_2$) receptors
e. serotonin (5-HT) receptors

**340.** A 27-year-old male has sprained his ankle, which is swollen and painful, while skiing. X-ray examination is negative except for the appearance of swelling. An NSAID is administered. Which of the following would be decreased?

a. histamine
b. cortisol
c. bradykinin
d. prostacyclin
e. uric acid

**341.** A 74-year-old female has had several episodes of transient ischemic attacks (TIAs). She cannot tolerate aspirin. Which of the following should be considered as an alternative therapy?

a. streptokinase
b. dipyridamole
c. acetaminophen
d. ticlopidine
e. aminocaproic acid

**342.** A 16-year-old female is brought to the emergency department (ED) because of increasing drowsiness and inattentiveness. Her family tells you that she takes medication for epilepsy and may have taken an extra dose that day. On examination, she has ataxic gait, nystagmus, and gingival hypertrophy. What medication does she take?

a. phenytoin
b. carbamazepine
c. ethosuximide
d. valproic acid
e. trimethadione

**343.** What is the "on-off phenomenon" associated with levodopa (L-dopa) therapy?

a. fluctuation in clinical response independent of drug levels
b. improvement of clinical response after a drug holiday
c. shortened duration of clinical response per dose

**344.** A 29-year-old female has a 10-year history of migraine headaches. She can usually sense onset. Which of the following agents is the drug of choice for countering acute onset of her headaches?

a. ergotamine   (Prophylaxis)
b. propranolol
c. methysergide
d. pseudoephedrine
e. aspirin

**345.** A common side effect of antihistamines is sedation. A newer antihistamine terfenadine, is often used because it is less sedating than traditional antihistamines; however, a dangerous drug-drug interaction can occur. What is it?

a. the combination of terfenadine and warfarin causes hemorrhaging
b. the combination of terfenadine and benzodiazepines causes respiratory depression
c. the combination of terfenadine and prazocin causes hypotension
d. the combination of terfenadine and erythromycin causes ventricular arrhythmias

**DIRECTIONS:** Each numbered question or incomplete statement is NEGATIVELY phrased. Select the **one best** lettered response.

**346.** A 65-year-old female has swelling and pain in several of the interphalangeal (IP) joints of her hand. X-ray examination reveals arthritic changes. Which agent should NOT be prescribed?

a. indomethacin
b. acetaminophen
c. tolmetin
d. naproxen
e. piroxicam

**347.** Which of the following H$_1$ receptor antagonists (antihistamines) causes the LEAST sedation at therapeutic doses?

a. hydroxyzine
b. diphenhydramine
c. terfenadine
d. promethazine
e. tripelennamine

**348.** Which adverse effect of L-dopa therapy is NOT improved by adding carbidopa?

a. mydriasis
b. cardiac arrhythmia
c. nausea
d. depression

**349.** All the following are therapeutic uses of natural prostaglandins or synthetic prostaglandin derivatives EXCEPT

a. abortion
b. cervical ripening in pregnant women
c. temporary maintenance of the patency of the ductus arteriosus in preterm neonates
d. prevention of gastric ulceration caused by nonsteroidal anti-inflammatory drugs
e. treatment of chronic obstructive pulmonary diseases like bronchial asthma

**350.** All the following are effects of serotonin (5-HT) EXCEPT

a. increased heart rate and force of contraction
b. vasoconstriction of arterioles of the pulmonary and renal beds
c. stimulation of pain and itching responses
d. contraction of bronchial smooth muscle
e. relaxation of gastrointestinal (GI) smooth muscle

# LOCAL CONTROL
# SUBSTANCES

## *Answers*

**336. The answer is e.** (*DiPalma, 4/e, pp 201–202. Katzung, 7/e, p 276.*) Sumatriptan is closely related to serotonin (5-HT) in structure, and it is believed that the drug is effective in the treatment of acute migraine headaches by virtue of its selective agonistic activity at 5-HT$_{1D}$ receptors. These receptors, present on cerebral and meningeal arteries, mediate vaso-constriction induced by 5-HT. In addition, 5-HT$_{1D}$ receptors are found on presynaptic nerve terminals and function to inhibit the release of neuropeptides and other neurotransmitters. It has been suggested that the pain of migraine headaches is caused by vasodilation of intracranial blood vessels and stimulation of trigeminovascular axons, which cause pain and release vasoactive neuropeptides to produce neurogenic inflammation and edema. Sumatriptan acts to reduce vasodilation and the release of neurotransmitters and, therefore, reduces the pain associated with migraine headaches. Other antimigraine drugs (e.g., ergotamine and dihydroergotamine) also exhibit high affinities for the 5-HT$_{1D}$ receptor site.

**337. The answer is a.** (*DiPalma, 4/e, pp 188–189. Katzung, 7/e, p 262.*) H$_1$ receptors appear to be linked to phospholipase C; activation of these receptors results in an increase in the intracellular formation of inositol-1,4,5-trisphosphate (IP$_3$) and 1,2-diacylglycerol. IP$_3$ binds to a receptor located on the endoplasmic reticulum, initiating the release of calcium (Ca) into the cytosol, where it activates Ca-dependent protein kinases. Diacylglycerol activates protein kinase C. Additionally, stimulation of H$_1$ receptors may activate phospholipase A$_2$ and trigger the arachidonic acid cascade, leading to prostaglandin production.

H$_2$ receptors are associated with adenylate cyclase and stimulation of these receptors increases the cytosolic concentration of cyclic AMP and activation of cyclic AMP-dependent protein kinase. Although inhibition of adenylate cyclase has been suggested as the intracellular signaling mechanism associated with H$_3$ receptors, this has not been completely substantiated.

**338. The answer is a.** *(DiPalma, 4/e, pp 345–353. Katzung, 7/e, pp 579–584.)* Aspirin (acetylsalicylic acid) is the most extensively used analgesic, antipyretic, and anti-inflammatory agent of the group of compounds known as *NSAIDs*, or *nonopioid analgesics*. Most of its therapeutic and adverse effects appear to be related to the inhibition of prostaglandin synthesis. NSAIDs inhibit the activity of the enzyme cyclooxygenase, which mediates the conversion of arachidonic acid to prostaglandins that are involved in pain, fever, and inflammation. Aspirin may produce irritation and ulceration of the GI tract, an adverse effect that is about equal to other salicylates. It also inhibits platelet aggregation. Acetaminophen, like aspirin, has analgesic and antipyretic properties but does not have clinically significant anti-inflammatory activity and is not irritating to the GI tract.

**339. The answer is c.** *(DiPalma, 4/e, p 203. Katzung, 7/e, p 227.)* Cyproheptadine is a potent antagonist at serotonin (5-HT) and histamine (H$_1$) receptors; in addition, high doses will block muscarinic receptor sites. The drug has no activity at H$_2$, adrenergic, dopaminergic, nicotinic, or benzodiazepine receptors. Clinically, cyproheptadine is used as an antihistamine for allergic conditions (e.g., allergic rhinitis, urticaria, pruritus). Because of its ability to inhibit the activity of 5-HT receptors, the drug is also useful in treating hypermotility of the GI tract associated with carcinoid tumors and in the prophylaxis of severe headaches in children.

**340. The answer is d.** *(Hardman and Limbird, 9/e, p 617. Katzung, 7/e, p 306.)* Most NSAIDs inhibit both cyclooxygenase I and II, resulting in decreased synthesis of prostaglandins, prostacyclins, and thromboxanes.

**341. The answer is d.** *(Hardman and Limbird, 9/e, p 1354. Katzung, 7/e, p 557.)* Ticlopidine decreases platelet aggregation by an unknown mechanism that inhibits binding of fibrinogen to activated platelets. Ticlopidine has no effect on prostaglandin synthesis.

**342. The answer is a.** *(Hardman and Limbird, 9/e, pp 469–470.)* Phenytoin has a narrow toxic-therapeutic range. Early signs of phenytoin toxicity are diplopia, nystagmus, and ataxia; sedation occurs at higher drug levels. Gingival hypertrophy, hirsutism, peripheral neuropathy, and folate-deficiency anemia can occur with long-term use. Phenytoin toxicity can be induced by drugs that displace it from plasma proteins.

**343. The answer is a.** (*Hardman and Limbird, 9/e, p 510. Katzung, 7/e, p 454.*) Fluctuations in clinical response to levodopa may or may not be related to drug levels (time of last dose). The likelihood of both kinds of fluctuation increases with longer duration of treatment. When these fluctuations are unrelated to drug levels, they are termed the "on-off phenomenon"; the mechanism is unclear.

**344. The answer is a.** (*DiPalma, 4/e, pp 202–203. Hardman and Limbird, 9/e, p 495.*) Ergotamine has several pharmacologic properties, including blockade of $\alpha$-adrenergic receptors; however, its mechanism of action in treating migraine headaches is primarily related to its agonistic interaction with serotonin receptors ($5\text{-HT}_{1D}$), resulting in vasoconstriction. Although chronic treatment with this nonsedative, nonanalgesic drug does not decrease the frequency of or prevent migraine attacks, an oral dose of ergotamine is the drug of choice for combating an incipient attack of migraine headache, especially during the prodromal stage.

**345. The answer is d.** (*Katzung, 7/e, pp 269–270, 999. Hardman and Limbird, 9/e, p 951.*) Erythromycin inhibits terfenadine metabolism. When terfenadine is taken in higher-than-recommended doses or when it is not efficiently metabolized, increased serum concentrations can cause cardiac arrhythmias. Terfenadine blocks delayed rectifier potassium (K) channels, resulting in prolongation of the QT interval and polymorphic ventricular tachycardia (VT).

**346. The answer is b.** (*DiPalma, 4/e, pp 347, 354–361. Hardman and Limbird, 9/e, pp 631–633.*) All of the drugs listed, except acetaminophen, are usually considered NSAIDs, a large group of structurally dissimilar compounds. These drugs share the pharmacologic properties of the prototype compound, aspirin, in that all have analgesic, antipyretic, and anti-inflammatory effects. The mechanism of action responsible for the effect of NSAIDs is reduction in the formation of eicosanoids (e.g., prostaglandins, thromboxanes) by inhibiting the enzyme cyclooxygenase. Acetaminophen differs from the other drugs in that it is a very weak anti-inflammatory agent; however, it is an effective analgesic and antipyretic.

**347. The answer is c.** (*DiPalma, 4/e, pp 193–194. Katzung, 7/e, p 265–268.*) As a group $H_1$-receptor antagonists elicit depressive effects on the CNS at therapeutic doses; thus, most of these compounds will cause varying degrees of diminished alertness, slowed reaction time, muscle weakness, mild sedation, and even somnolence. Some of the drugs are more likely to produce these CNS manifestations than others, and patients seem to vary in susceptibility and responsiveness. The aminoalkyl ethers are especially liable to produce sedation; for example, diphenhydramine can produce drowsiness in 20 to 50% of patients.

In some circumstances, physicians may take advantage of this sedative effect by using one of these drugs as a sedative prior to or after surgery or may prescribe an $H_1$-receptor antagonist for patients who are having problems sleeping. For example, hydroxyzine and promethazine are indicated for preoperative and postoperative sedation, and diphenhydramine is contained in most over-the-counter (OTC) preparations that aid in sleeping. Tripelennamine, used in patients with allergic rhinitis and other allergies, may cause significant drowsiness in some patients.

Some of the newer antihistamines (e.g., terfenadine, astemizole, loratadine) elicit reduced or minimal sedative effects. For the most part, these drugs do not cross the blood-brain barrier very well at effective therapeutic doses and, therefore, produce a low incidence of CNS effects.

**348. The answer is d.** (*Katzung, 7/e, pp 451–455.*) Adding carbidopa decreases the amount of dopamine (DM) formed peripherally from dopa by dopa decarboxylase. Depression, psychosis, and other psychiatric adverse effects of L-dopa are mediated by CNS DM, so adding carbidopa does not make them less likely. The combination of L-dopa and carbidopa reduces the extracerebral metabolism of L-dopa, resulting in decreased peripheral adverse effects.

**349. The answer is e.** (*DiPalma, 4/e, pp 214–215.*) Because they stimulate uterine contraction, both dinoprostone (prostaglandin $E_2$) [$PGE_2$]) and carboprost (15-methyl-prostaglandin $F_{2\alpha}$ [15-methyl-$PGF_{2\alpha}$]) are available for use as abortifacients. Typically, dinoprostone (administered by vaginal suppository) and 15-methyl-$PGF_{2\alpha}$ (given by intramuscular [IM] injection) are used for therapeutic abortions between the 12th and 20th weeks of gestation. In addition, dinoprostone can be used up to the 28th gestational week when intrauterine fetal death has occurred. Dinoprostone is also indicated for cervical ripening (softening, effacement, and dilation) in pregnant women at or near term who present with a medical or obstetric need to have labor induced; for this purpose, the drug (as a gel) is introduced directly into the cervical canal.

(c) Alprostadil (prostaglandin $E_1$ [$PGE_1$]) is used therapeutically in preterm infants to temporarily maintain the patency of the ductus arteriosus until corrective surgery can be performed. The drug is administered by continuous intravenous infusion or by catheter through the umbilical artery and should only be used in pediatric intensive care facilities. Misoprostol is a synthetic analogue of $PGE_1$ (15-deoxy-16-hydroxy-16-methyl-$PGE_1$ methyl ester). It is indicated for the prevention of gastric ulcers in patients taking nonsteroidal anti-inflammatory drugs (e.g., aspirin, indomethacin) and is administered orally.

Some prostaglandins, especially $PGE_1$, $PGE_2$, and $PGI_2$ (prostacyclin), are potent bronchodilators and many prostaglandin analogues have been tested for use in chronic obstructive pulmonary disease. Unfortunately prostaglandins are irritating to the airways and cause coughing when inhaled, which has precluded their use as antiasthmatic drugs. A number of leukotriene (LT) antagonists, however, are being examined clinically for use in the treatment of diseases such as bronchial asthma.

( MONTELEUKOSTAT )  In Use

**350.   The answer is e.** (*DiPalma, 4/e, pp 199–201. Katzung, 7/e, pp 274–276.*) In the periphery, serotonin (5-HT) exerts many effects on a variety of tissues. The effects of this endogenous amine are mediated through an array of 5-HT receptor subtypes and are species-dependent and variable, making it difficult to generalize. However, in humans all the effects described in the question may occur following exogenous administration of this substance except for relaxation of GI smooth muscle. The enterochromaffin cells of the intestine contain about 90% of the body's stores of 5-HT. The amine causes GI smooth muscle to contract by both a direct action on 5-HT receptors of the muscle and by stimulation of parasympathetic ganglia found within the intestinal wall. Although it is believed that 5-HT serves a physiologic function by increasing tone and facilitating peristalsis, it may also be involved in certain diseases (e.g., carcinoid tumor) in which an overproduction of 5-HT results in diarrhea.

# RENAL SYSTEM

**Note: In the classification of drugs, prototype drugs are marked with an asterisk (*).**

Carbonic Anhydrase Inhibitors
  Acetazolamide*
Loop Diuretics
  Bumetanide
  Ethacrynic acid
  Furosemide*
  Torsemide
Osmotic Diuretics
  Mannitol
Potassium (K)-Sparing Diuretics
  Amiloride
  Spironolactone*
  Triamterene*

Thiazide (Benzodiathiazide) Diuretics
  Bendroflumethiazide
  Chlorothiazide*
  Hydrochlorothiazide
  Polythiazide
Thiazide-Related Compounds
  Chlorthalidone
  Indapamide
  Metolazone
Antidiuretic Hormone
  Vasopressin*
  Desmopressin
  Lypressin

175

# Questions

**DIRECTIONS:** Each question below contains several suggested responses. Select the **one best** response to each question.

**351.** The structure shown below is a member of which of the following drug groups?

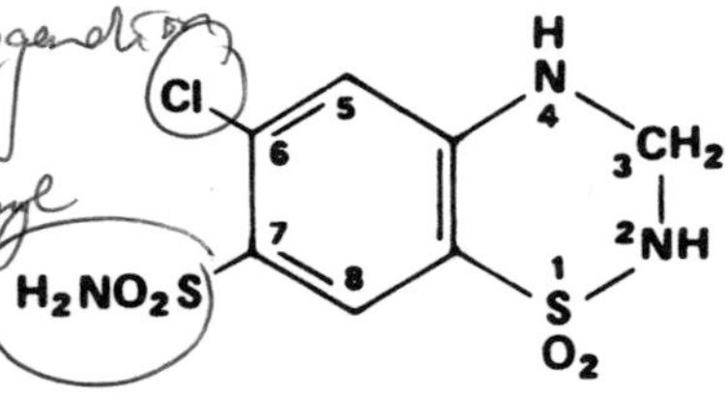

*[handwritten annotations: (a) Halogens, (b) Sulfonyl group, with circles around "Cl" and "H₂NO₂S"]*

a. osmotic diuretics
b. loop diuretics
c. thiazide diuretics
d. K-sparing diuretics
e. carbonic anhydrase inhibitors

**352.** Torsemide inhibits the sodium-potassium-dichloride ($Na^+/K^+/2Cl^-$) cotransporters that are located in the

*[handwritten: loop]*

a. collecting duct
b. ascending limb of the loop of Henle
d. descending limb of the loop of Henle
d. proximal tubule
e. distal convoluted tubule

**353.** Canrenone, which elicits a diuretic response, is a major biotransformation product of which of the following agents?

a. indapamide
b. chlorthalidone
c. spironolactone
d. amiloride
e. triamterene

**354.** Hyperkalemia is a contraindication to the use of which of the following drugs?

a. acetazolamide
b. chlorothiazide
c. ethacrynic acid
d. chlorthalidone
e. spironolactone

**355.** A reduction in insulin release from the pancreas may be caused by which of the following diuretics?

a. triamterene
b. chlorothiazide
c. spironolactone
d. acetazolamide
e. amiloride

*[handwritten notes at bottom right]*

*(Tumonz lysis Syndrome)*

*Steroid Nucleus*

**356.** Acute uric acid nephropathy, which is characterized by the acute overproduction of uric acid and by extreme hyperuricemia, can best be prevented with

a. antidiuretic hormone (ADH) (vasopressin [VP])
b. cyclophosphamide
c. allopurinol
d. amiloride
e. sodium chloride (NaCl)

**357.** The release of ADH is suppressed by which of the following drugs to promote a diuresis?

a. guanethidine
b. acetazolamide
c. chlorothiazide
d. ethanol
e. indomethacin

**358.** Conservation of K ions in the body occurs with which of the following diuretics?

a. furosemide
b. hydrochlorothiazide
c. triamterene
d. metolazone
e. bumetanide

*repeat O*

**359.** Spironolactone can be characterized by which one of the following statements?

a. it is biotransformed to an inactive product
b. it binds to a cytoplasmic receptor
c. it is a more potent diuretic than is hydrochlorothiazide
d. it interferes with aldosterone synthesis
e. it inhibits Na reabsorption in the proximal renal tubule of the nephron

**360.** An enhancement of the parathyroid hormone-mediated reabsorption of calcium (Ca) in the distal tubule is caused by which of the following diuretics?

a. acetazolamide
b. furosemide
c. triamterene
d. bumetanide
e. hydrochlorothiazide

$PTH$ / Phosphaturic
$\downarrow$    Acn
$\uparrow$ $Ca^{2+}$ reabsorption

**DIRECTIONS:** Each numbered question or incomplete statement below is NEGATIVELY phrased. Select the **one best** lettered response.

**361.** Mannitol may be useful in all the following procedures EXCEPT

a.  treatment of elevated intracranial pressure
b.  treatment of elevated intraocular pressure
c.  treatment of pulmonary edema with congestive heart failure (CHF)
d.  diagnostic evaluation of acute oliguria
e.  prophylaxis of acute renal failure

**362.** When furosemide is administered concomitantly with other drugs, all the following can occur EXCEPT

a.  reduction of renal clearance of lithium
b.  enhancement of ototoxicity of gentamicin
c.  reduction of renal excretion of salicylates
d.  augmentation of pressor action of norepinephrine
e.  attenuation of neuromuscular blocking effect of tubocurarine

**363.** Adverse interactions may occur between thiazides and all the following drug groups EXCEPT

a.  adrenal corticosteroids
b.  anticoagulants (oral)
c.  aminoglycosides
d.  β-adrenergic blockers
e.  antidepolarizing skeletal muscle relaxants

**364.** Diuretic agents that indirectly cause an increased binding of digoxin to cardiac tissue sodium-potassium-adenosine triphosphatase ($Na^+/K^+/ATPase$) include all the following EXCEPT

a.  hydrochlorothiazide
b.  torsemide
c.  amiloride
d.  ethacrynic acid
e.  indapamide

**365.** Properties of mannitol include all the following EXCEPT

a.  retention of water in the tubular fluid
b.  the ability to be metabolically altered to an active form
c.  the capacity to be freely filtered
d.  effectiveness as nonelectrolytic, osmotically active particles
e.  the ability to resist complete reabsorption by the renal tubule

**366.** True statements about adverse reactions that apply to both hydrochlorothiazide and torsemide include all the following EXCEPT

a.  they may produce hyperglycemia
b.  they elevate blood levels of uric acid
c.  they decrease blood pressure
d.  they may cause hyperlipidemia
e.  they lower serum levels of magnesium (Mg)

**367.** Adverse reactions associated with furosemide include all the following EXCEPT

a.  hyperglycemia
b.  tinnitus
c.  fluid and electrolyte imbalance
d.  hypotension
e.  metabolic acidosis

**368.** Adverse reactions associated with both acetazolamide and antibacterial sulfonamides include all the following EXCEPT

a.  formation of urinary calculi
b.  fever
c.  metabolic acidosis
d.  crystalluria
e.  exfoliative dermatitis

**369.** Hydrochlorothiazide is clinically useful in the treatment of all the following EXCEPT

a.  edema caused by CHF
b.  edema induced by glucocorticoids
c.  hypertension with or without edema
d.  liver disease with ascites
e.  glaucoma by reduction of intraocular pressure

/ acetylamide - Met. Acidosis

**DIRECTIONS:** Each group of questions below consists of lettered headings followed by a set of numbered items. For each numbered item select the **one** lettered heading with which it is **most** closely associated. Each lettered heading may be used **once, more than once, or not at all.**

### Questions 370–372

The figure below shows proposed sites of action of drugs. For each of the diuretic agents below, choose the anatomic site in the schematic diagram of the renal nephron where the principal action of the agent occurs.

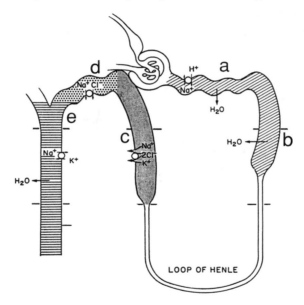

(Modified from *DiPalma, 4/e,* with permission.)

C **370.** ethacrynic acid *(loop Diuretics)*

d **371.** indapamide *(thiazide-related)*

e **372.** triamterene *(k⁺ sparing)*

## Questions 373–375

The table below shows the urinary excretion patterns of electrolytes of diuretic drugs. For each of the diuretic agents listed below, choose the urinary excretion pattern that the drug would produce.

| Drug | $Na^+$ | $Cl^-$ | $K^+$ | $Ca^{2+}$ | $HCO_3^-$ | $Mg^{2+}$ |
|------|------|------|------|------|------|------|
| a. | + | + | + | − | ± | + |
| b. | + | + | + | − | 0 | + |
| c. | + | + | + | + | 0 | + |
| d. | + | + | − | 0 | + | 0 |
| e. | + | − | + | 0 | + | 0 |

+ = increase; − = decrease; 0 = no change; ± = increase dependent on dose

**373.** triamterene

**374.** torsemide

**375.** bumetanide

## Questions 376–378

Match each statement with the appropriate drug.

a. metolazone
b. ethacrynic acid
c. chlorthalidone
d. triamterene
e. spironolactone
f. acetazolamide
g. furosemide
h. mannitol
i. amiloride
j. hydrochlorothiazide

**376.** The urinary excretion of chloride ($Cl^-$) is decreased

**377.** Elevated intraocular and cerebrospinal fluid pressures are reduced

**378.** Chemically, this compound is a steroid

# RENAL SYSTEM

## Answers

**351. The answer is c.** (*DiPalma, 4/e, pp 457–458, 463–464. Hardman and Limbird, 9/e, p 703.*) The structure shown in the question is hydrochlorothiazide and is one of several of the thiazide (benzothiadiazide) diuretics. Halogenation of the benzothiadiazine ring at C 6 and a free sulfamyl group ($-SO_2NH_2$) at C 7 are necessary for maximal diuretic activity in the series of compounds. In contrast to the carbonic anhydrase inhibitors, benzothiadiazides can act independently of acid-base balance. An example of an osmotic diuretic is mannitol; representatives of the loop diuretics are furosemide, ethacrynic acid, and bumetanide. Potassium-sparing diuretics are spironolactone (a steroid), triamterene (a pteridine derivative), and amiloride (a pyrazinecarbonyl-guanidine).

**352. The answer is b.** (*DiPalma, 4/e, pp 455–456, 460–462.*) Torsemide is a loop diuretic that promotes the urinary excretion of Na and $Cl^-$. This diuretic agent blocks the reabsorption of Na and $Cl^-$ by inhibiting the $Na^+/K^+/2Cl^-$ cotransporters in the ascending limb of the loop of Henle. Although this cotransport mechanism requires energy from converting adenosine triphosphate (ATP) to adenosine diphosphate (ADP) by $Na^+,K^+$-ATPase, torsemide does not directly inhibit the enzyme $Na^+/K^+/ATPase$. Along with the net loss of Na and $Cl^-$, loop diuretics produce an increase in the urinary excretion of Ca and Mg by interfering with the reabsorption of these ions in the ascending limb of the loop of Henle. In addition, torsemide, like the other loop diuretic agents, can cause hypokalemia. The secretion of the K occurs as a consequence of the reabsorption of Na in the late distal convoluted tubule and the collecting duct. The diuretic effect of torsemide has a duration of 6 to 8 h.

**353. The answer is c.** (*DiPalma, 4/e, pp 463–464. Hardman and Limbird, 9/e, p 708.*) Canrenone is the active biotransformation product of spironolactone. Similar to spironolactone, it is a competitive antagonist of aldosterone in the collecting duct of the nephron. Canrenone, like spironolactone, can bind to the cytoplasmic aldosterone receptor and prevent the receptor from being converted to the active conformation. Since the active conformation is prevented, reduction of NaCl reabsorption and K retention results. The diuretic action of spironolactone is partially due to the presence of canrenone. Indapamide, chlorthalidone, amiloride, and furosemide are not biotransformed to active products. Triamterene, however, is converted to some products that exhibit diuretic activity.

**354. The answer is e.** *(DiPalma, 4/e, pp 463–464. Hardman and Limbird, 9/e, p 708.)* Spironolactone is a competitive antagonist of aldosterone that blocks the reabsorption of Na and water from the collecting duct in exchange for K and hydrogen ion retention. Therefore, in the presence of hyperkalemia, spironolactone is contraindicated. The administration of each of the other diuretic agents listed in the question results in increased excretion of K.

**355. The answer is b.** *(DiPalma, 4/e, pp 458–459, 461–462. Hardman and Limbird, 9/e, pp 702–704.)* An adverse reaction reported to occur occasionally with the thiazides, such as chlorothiazide, is hyperglycemia. In addition, hyperglycemia may occur with thiazide-related compounds (chlorthalidone and metolazone) and the high-ceiling diuretics (ethacrynic acid, furosemide, and bumetanide). The proposed mechanism for the elevation in blood glucose appears to be related to a decrease in insulin release from the pancreas. In addition increased glycogenolysis, decreased glycogenesis, and a reduction in the conversion of proinsulin to insulin may also be involved in the hyperglycemic response. Diazoxide, a nondiuretic thiazide, is given to treat hypoglycemia in certain conditions. However, diazoxide is used more often to control hypertensive emergencies.

**356. The answer is c.** *(DiPalma, 4/e, pp 362–363, 660. Hardman and Limbird, 9/e, pp 649–650.)* Acute hyperuricemia, which often occurs in patients treated with cytotoxic drugs for neoplasic disorders, can lead to the deposition of urate crystals in the kidneys and their collecting ducts. This can produce partial or complete obstruction of the collecting ducts, renal pelvis, or ureter. Allopurinol and its primary metabolite, alloxanthine, are inhibitors of xanthine oxidase, an enzyme that catalyzes the oxidation of hypoxanthine and xanthine to uric acid. The use of allopurinol in patients at risk can markedly reduce the likelihood that they will develop acute uric acid nephropathy.

**357. The answer is d.** *(DiPalma, 4/e, pp 256, 457, 465.)* Ethanol produces a diuretic response by inhibiting the release of antidiuretic hormone (ADH)

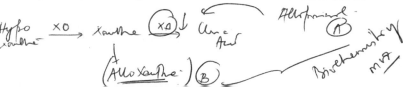

from the posterior pituitary gland. Less antidiuretic hormone acts on the collecting duct of the nephron and, therefore, the amount of water reabsorbed by the collecting duct is reduced. Indomethacin enhances the release of antidiuretic hormone, which increases the permeability of the collecting duct to water. Acetazolamide and chlorothiazide promote a diuresis by acting on a site directly in the nephron unit to reduce the reabsorption of NaCl and water. Guanethidine, an antihypertensive agent, does not appear to alter the release of antidiuretic hormone.

**358.  The answer is c.** (*DiPalma, 4/e, pp 457–464. Hardman and Limbird, 9/e, pp 704–706.*) Triamterene produces retention of the K ion by inhibiting in the collecting duct the reabsorption of Na, which is accompanied by the excretion of K ions. The loop diuretics furosemide and bumetanide cause as a possible adverse action the development of hypokalemia. In addition, thiazides (e.g., hydrochlorothiazide) and the thiazide-related agents (e.g., metolazone) can cause the loss of K ions with the consequences of hypokalemia. Triamterene is generally given with a loop diuretic or thiazide to prevent or correct the condition of hypokalemia.

**359.  The answer is b.** (*DiPalma, 4/e, pp 463–464. Hardman and Limbird, 9/e, pp 706–709.*) Spironolactone is a K-sparing diuretic. The drug is well absorbed from the gastrointestinal tract and is biotransformed in the liver to an active metabolite, canrenone. Spironolactone is contraindicated in the presence of hyperkalemia, since this aldosterone antagonist may cause further elevation of plasma K concentrations. It does not appear to depress adrenal or pituitary function. CNS side effects of the drug can include lethargy, headache, drowsiness, and mental confusion. Spironolactone displaces aldosterone from receptor sites that are responsible for Na resorption in the collecting duct of the nephron; it does not interfere with the synthesis of aldosterone.

**360.  The answer is e.** (*DiPalma, 4/e, pp 456–458, 460.*) In the distal tubule of the nephron Na and $Cl^-$ ions are reabsorbed. In addition, Ca ions are reabsorbed by a parathyroid-mediated response. Thiazide diuretics (e.g., hydrochlorothiazide) have their site of action on the distal tubule and inhibit the reabsorption of Na and $Cl^-$ but enhance the parathyroid-mediated increase of Ca reabsorption. The urinary excretion of Na and $Cl^-$ is increased, while excretion of Ca is reduced. Loop diuretics such as furosemide and bumetanide increase the urinary excretion of Ca ions and may be used in the treatment of acute hypercalcemia. Acetazolamide and triamterene do not appear to inhibit the reabsorption of Ca ions in the distal tubule.

**361. The answer is c.** (*DiPalma, 4/e, p 466. Hardman and Limbird, 9/e, pp 695–697.*) Mannitol increases serum osmolarity and therefore "pulls" water out of cells, cerebrospinal fluid, and aqueous humor. This effect can be useful in the treatment of elevated intraocular or intracranial pressure. However, by expanding the intravascular volume, mannitol can exacerbate CHF. Mannitol will increase urine output if oliguria is caused by a decreased glomerular filtration rate but not if the oliguria is secondary to tubular dysfunction. Mannitol is useful in the prevention of acute renal failure as a means of maintaining an adequate flow of relatively dilute urine.

**362. The answer is d.** (*DiPalma, 4/e, p 462.*) The diuretic agents are involved in a number of interactions when they are given concomitantly with another drug. The loop diuretic furosemide is an example of this class of drugs that can cause several drug-drug interactions. Furosemide can enhance the toxicity of lithium by reducing its renal excretion. Since the loop diuretic can cause hearing impairment, it can augment the ototoxicity that can occur with other drugs, such as aminoglycoside antibiotics (e.g., gentamicin, streptomycin, tobramycin). Furosemide undergoes proximal tubule secretion. This renal secretory mechanism, which is associated with renal excretion, is also available to a number of organic acids, such as the salicylates. When salicylates are present in the body, furosemide is a competitive inhibitor of their excretion by this particular mechanism in the proximal tubule; therefore, the plasma levels of salicylates are increased with the potential for adverse reactions in the patient. Interactions between norepinephrine and furosemide have been reported. The hypertensive effect of norepinephrine is decreased when it is administered with furosemide. Furosemide should be discontinued in a patient prior to surgery. This diuretic agent may also reduce the skeletal muscle relaxant effects of tubocurarine.

**363. The answer is c.** (*AMA Drug Evaluations Annual, 1993, p 692. DiPalma, 4/e, pp 458–459.*) Drug interactions are reported for various drugs and the thiazide diuretics. Thiazides can indirectly promote the loss of K from the collecting duct of the nephron, and adrenal corticosteroids can enhance the hypokalemic effect. The therapeutic effect of oral anticoagulants may be reduced by thiazides because these diuretics can concentrate clotting factors in the blood. Thiazide diuretics elevate blood lipid, urate, and glucose levels and these effects can be augmented in the presence of a β-adrenergic blocker. In addition, the neuromuscular blocking action of tubocurarine is enhanced by thiazide diuretics. Aminoglycosides, which can cause eighth nerve damage, can increase the ototoxicity that is associated with the use of the loop diuretics. Tinnitus and ototoxicity have not been reported as adverse reactions for the thiazide diuretics.

**364. The answer is c.** (*DiPalma, 4/e, pp 458, 461, 464.*) Diuretic therapy can lead to the development of hypokalemia. The thiazides (hydrochlorothiazide), thiazide-related compounds (indapamide), and loop diuretics (ethacrynic acid, torsemide) can produce the loss of K from the blood through the late distal tubule and collecting duct into the renal tubular fluid. When any of these drugs are administered in the presence of digitalis glycoside (digoxin), there is the potential for digitalis toxicities to occur. The development of these toxicities is related to the fact that in the presence of hypokalemia there is greater affinity of digitalis glycosides to cardiac tissue $Na^+/K^+/ATPase$. However, when the hypokalemia is corrected and the plasma levels of K are returned toward normal, digitalis toxicities are usually eliminated. Amiloride, which is a K-sparing diuretic, does not cause hypokalemia and, therefore, would not enhance the binding of digoxin to $Na^+/K^+/ATPase$. As a matter of fact, amiloride promotes the conservation of K and can cause the adverse reaction of hyperkalemia.

**365. The answer is b.** (*DiPalma, 4/e, p 466. Hardman and Limbird, 9/e, pp 695–697.*) A significant increase in the amount of any osmotically active solute in voided urine is usually accompanied by an increase in urine volume. Osmotic diuretics effect diuresis through this principle. The osmotic diuretics (such as mannitol) are nonelectrolytes that are freely filtered at the glomerulus, undergo limited reabsorption by the renal tubules, retain water in the renal tubule, and promote an osmotic diuresis, generally without significant Na excretion. In addition, these diuretics resist alteration by metabolic processes.

**366. The answer is d.** (*DiPalma, 4/e, pp 458, 461–462.*) The thiazide diuretics and the loop diuretics have a number of adverse reactions in common. Hydrochlorothiazide and the loop diuretic torsemide cause hyperglycemia by possibly reducing the secretion of insulin from the pancreas. Since these drugs can elevate blood levels of glucose they should be used with caution when administered to patients with diabetes mellitus. The development of hyperuricemia as a consequence of the use of hydrochlorothiazide or torsemide is related to the fact that these drugs interfere with the proximal tubule secretion of uric acid and cause volume depletion. Neither torsemide nor hydrochlorothiazide has any effect on the synthesis of uric acid. Both hydrochlorothiazide and torsemide are indicated in the treatment of hypertension. These drugs will bring about a reduction in elevated blood pressure. This effect is considered an adverse reaction if it occurs when the drugs are employed as diuretic agents to remove edematous fluid from a patient. Of the diuretic agents only the thiazide drugs have been reported to cause an elevation in blood lipids (hyperlipidemia). The mechanism of action for this effect on lipids is unknown. The alteration in serum Mg (hypomagnesemia) is caused by both hydrochlorothiazide and torsemide. These diuretic agents block the reabsorption of Mg.

**367. The answer is e.** *(DiPalma, 4/e, pp 460–462. Hardman and Limbird, 9/e, pp 697–701.)* The loop, or high-ceiling, diuretics furosemide and ethacrynic acid are cleared by the kidney with such celerity that even high doses repeatedly administered do not result in significant accumulation. Chronic administration of these agents, however, may lead to alkalosis with hyponatremia in association with rapid removal of edema fluid. Other toxic manifestations of loop diuretics include fluid and electrolyte imbalance, gastrointestinal symptoms, interstitial nephritis, hyperglycemia, tinnitus, and infrequent, but serious, ototoxicity. Besides being used as a diuretic agent, furosemide is used in the treatment of hypertension.

**368. The answer is c.** *(DiPalma, 4/e, p 465. Katzung, 7/e, pp 246–249.)* Acetazolamide, an aromatic sulfonamide derivative, is a mild diuretic agent that increases the loss of Na and water from the body by inhibiting the enzyme carbonic anhydrase. The sulfonamides, a group of antibacterial agents, exert their antimicrobial effect on Gram-positive and Gram-negative bacteria by competitive antagonism of para-aminobenzoic acid (PABA). Acetazolamide and the sulfonamides are reported to have some similar adverse reactions. Fever, blood dyscrasias, exfoliative dermatitis, skin rash, crystalluria, and formation of calculi may occur with the administration of either. Metabolic acidosis is associated only with the use of acetazolamide. Since this diuretic inhibits carbonic anhydrase in the proximal tubule, plasma levels of bicarbonate decrease, and if the reduction of bicarbonate is significant, metabolic acidosis can develop.

**369. The answer is e.** (*DiPalma, 4/e, pp 459, 465.*) Thiazides are most useful as diuretic agents in the management of edema caused by chronic cardiac decompensation. In the treatment of hypertensive disease, even without obvious edema, thiazides exert a hypotensive action that has proved beneficial. Less common uses of thiazide diuretics include the treatment of edema from glucocorticoids, diabetes insipidus, and hypercalciuria. The carbonic anhydrase inhibitor acetazolamide, by inhibiting the secretion of aqueous humor, has the property of decreasing intraocular pressure—an effect of value for patients who have glaucoma. Furosemide is the diuretic agent generally employed to treat acute pulmonary edema, although ethacrynic acid would be effective.

**370–372. The answers are 370-c, 371-d, 372-e.** (*DiPalma, 4/e, pp 456–466. Hardman and Limbird, 9/e, pp 697, 701, 705.*) The loop diuretic ethacrynic acid has its site of action in the ascending limb of the loop of Henle. This drug inhibits the reabsorption of Na and $Cl^-$ by interfering with the $Na^+/K^+/2Cl^-$ cotransport system. In addition, loop diuretics block the reabsorption of Mg and Ca from the renal tubular fluid into the blood in this segment of the nephron unit.

Indapamide, which is a thiazide-related compound, has its proposed site of action at the distal convoluted tubule or more specifically at the early portion of the distal tubule. The distal convoluted tubule is also the site of action for the thiazide diuretic agents (chlorothiazide, hydrochlorothiazide). Indapamide and hydrochlorothiazide inhibit the reabsorption of Na and $Cl^-$. These diuretics also promote the reabsorption of Ca back into the blood, but inhibit the reabsorption of Mg from the renal tubular fluid.

The K-sparing diuretic agents (spironolactone, triamterene, and amiloride) have their site of action in the nephron at the late distal tubule and the collecting duct. These diuretic agents only cause a mild natriuretic effect.

**373–375. The answers are 373-d, 374-c, 375-c.** (*DiPalma, 4/e, pp 457, 458, 460, 463–466.*) The urinary excretion pattern of electrolytes for the thiazide diuretic agents (e.g., chlorothiazide) shown in the table that accompanies the question is represented by choice a. These drugs block the reabsorption of Na and $Cl^-$ at the early distal convoluted tubule of the nephron. In addition, they promote the excretion of K and Mg. At high doses the thiazide diuretics (especially chlorothiazide) may cause a slight increase in bicarbonate excretion. As for the Ca ion, the thiazide diuretic agents enhance the distal tubular reabsorption of Ca, and, therefore, Ca urinary excretion may decrease.

The thiazide-related compounds (chlorthalidone, metolazone, indapamide) cause the same urinary excretion pattern of electrolytes but do not produce any change in bicarbonate excretion, since these drugs do not have the ability to inhibit carbonic anhydrase. The thiazide-related drugs are represented by choice b.

The loop diuretics (torsemide, bumetanide, furosemide, ethacrynic acid) are the most potent group of diuretic agents, and they are represented by choice c. These drugs act at the ascending limb of the loop of Henle and interfere with the cotransport of Na and Cl$^-$. In addition, they cause the excretion of K, Mg, and Ca into the urine.

The K-sparing group of diuretic agents are represented by choice d. Triamterene produces its diuretic response by reduction of the reabsorption of Na in the later distal convoluted tubule and the collecting duct. It causes an increase in the urinary excretion of NaCl and possibly bicarbonate, while it reduces the excretion of K. The K-sparing diuretic agents do not appear to have any significant effect on the excretion of Mg and Ca ions.

**376–378. The answers are 376-f, 377-h, 378-e.** (*DiPalma, 4/e, pp 463, 465–466. Hardman and Limbird, 9/e, 691, 693, 695–696, 707–708.*) Acetazolamide is a carbonic anhydrase inhibitor with its primary site of action at the proximal tubule of the nephron. Acetazolamide promotes a urinary excretion of Na, K, and bicarbonate. There is a decrease in loss of Cl$^-$ ions. The increased excretion of bicarbonate makes the urine alkaline and may produce metabolic acidosis as a consequence of the loss of bicarbonate from the blood. None of the other diuretic drugs promote a reduction in the excretion of the Cl$^-$ ion.

The only diuretic agent that has a steroid structure is spironolactone. This K-sparing diuretic is a competitive inhibitor of aldosterone, which mediates the reabsorption of Na ions in the collecting duct.

Mannitol is classified as an osmotic diuretic. It is used to maintain urine flow in such cases as trauma and drug intoxication as well as after surgery. In addition, mannitol is used to reduce pressure and volume of cerebrospinal fluid and pre- and postoperatively for short-term reduction of intraocular pressure. Although acetazolamide is used in the treatment of glaucoma, it is not employed to decrease cerebrospinal fluid pressure.

# GASTROINTESTINAL SYSTEM AND NUTRITION

Antacids *MCQ*
  Sodium (Na) bicarbonate
  Aluminum (Al) hydroxide
  Magnesium (Mg) hydroxide
  Calcium (Ca) carbonate
Histamine$_2$ (H$_2$)-Receptor Antagonists
  Cimetidine
  Ranitidine
  Famotidine
  Nizatidine
Proton-Pump Inhibitors
  Omeprazole
Mucosal Protective Agents
  Sucralfate
  Colloidal bismuth compounds–
  Bismuth subsalicylate
  Prostaglandins–misoprostol
  Promotion of Gastrointestinal
    (GI) Motility
  Metoclopramide
  Bethanechol
  Cisapride
Pancreatic Replacement Enzymes
  Pancrelipase (Pancrease,
    Cotazyme)
Laxatives *MCQ*
  Castor oil
  Cascara, senna, aloes, phenol-
    phthalein, bisacodyl
  Stool softeners
    Mineral oil, glycerine supposi-

tories, dioctyl sodium sulfosuc-
  cinate (docusate)
Bulk laxatives
  Hydrophilic colloids
  Saline cathartics
Antidiarrheal Drugs
  Diphenoxylate, loperamide *MCQ*
Dissolution of Gallstones
  Chenodeoxycholic acid
  Ursodiol (ursodeoxycholic acid)
Chronic Inflammatory Bowel
  Disease Sulfasalazine
Portal System Encephalopathy
  Lactulose
  Branched-chain amino acids
Vitamins
  Water-soluble    B & C
  Thiamine (B$_1$)
  Riboflavin (B$_2$)
  Nicotinic acid (NA; niacin)
  Pyridoxine (B$_6$)
  Vitamin C (ascorbic acid)
  Vitamin B$_{12}$
  Folic acid
  Fat-Soluble
  Vitamin A
  Vitamin D
  Vitamin E
  Vitamin K
Concept of recommended daily
  allowances (RDAs)

# Questions

**DIRECTIONS:** Each question below contains several suggested responses. Select the **one best** response to each question.

**379.** Cimetidine slows the metabolism of many drugs because it inhibits the activity of

a. monoamine oxidase (MAO)
b. cytochrome P-450
c. tyrosine kinase
d. hydrogen-potassium-adenosine triphosphatase (H+/K+/ATPase)
e. phase II glucoronidation reactions

**380.** The absorption of phosphate is reduced when large and prolonged doses of which of the following antacids are given?

a. Na bicarbonate
b. Mg hydroxide
c. Mg trisilicate
d. Ca carbonate
e. Sucralfate

**381.** Omeprazole, a new agent for the promotion of healing of peptic ulcers, has a mechanism of action based on

a. prostaglandins
b. gastric secretion
c. pepsin secretion
d. H+/K+/ATPase
e. anticholinergic action

**382.** An effective antidiarrheal agent that inhibits peristaltic movement is

a. clonidine
b. bismuth subsalicylate
c. oral electrolyte solution
d. atropine
e. diphenoxylate

**383.** The approved indication for misoprostol

a. reflux esophagitis
b. healing of gastric ulcer
c. healing of duodenal ulcer
d. prevention of gastric ulceration in patients using large doses of aspirin-like drugs
e. pathologic hypersecretory conditions such as Zollinger-Ellison syndrome

**384.** Metoclopramide has antiemetic properties because it

a. accelerates gastric emptying time
b. lowers esophageal sphincter pressure
c. is a central nervous system (CNS) dopamine (DM) receptor antagonist
d. has cholinomimetic properties
e. has sedative properties

**385.** The steatorrhea of pancreatic insufficiency can best be treated by

a. cimetidine
b. misoprostol
c. bile salts
d. pancrelipase
e. secretin

**386.** Cholesterol gallstones may be dissolved by oral treatment with

a. lovastatin
b. dehydrocholic acid
c. methyl tertiary butyl ether
d. chenodeoxycholic acid
e. monoctanoin

**387.** A drug of choice in the therapy of inflammatory bowel disease is

a. sulfadiazine
b. sulfasalazine
c. sulfapyridine
d. sulfamethoxazole
e. salicylate sodium

**388.** An important drug in the therapy of portal systemic encephalopathy is

a. lactulose
b. lactate
c. loperamide
d. lorazepam
e. loxapine

**389.** Bismuth salts are thought to be effective in peptic ulcer disease because they have bactericidal properties against

a. *Escherichia coli*
b. *Bacteroides fragilis*
c. *Clostridium difficile*
d. *Helicobacter pylori*
e. *Staphylococcus aureus*

**390.** Misoprostol has a cytoprotective action on the GI mucosa because it

a. enhances secretion of mucus and bicarbonate ion
b. neutralizes acid secretion
c. antagonizes nonsteroidal anti-inflammatory drugs (NSAIDs)
d. relieves ulcer symptoms
e. coats the mucosa

**391.** For the severe form of nodulocystic acne vulgaris, the first line of therapy is the systemic use of

a. vitamin A
b. retinol
c. tetracycline
d. isotretinoin (13-*cis*-retinoic acid)
e. ciprofloxacin

**392.** The primary pharmacologic action of omeprazole is reduction of

a. volume of gastric juice
b. gastric motility
c. secretion of pepsin
d. secretion of gastric acid
e. secretion of intrinsic factor

**393.** Which of the following vitamins in large doses is teratogenic?

a.  vitamin A
b.  vitamin $B_{12}$
c.  vitamin C
d.  vitamin D
e.  vitamin E

**394.** Fat-soluble vitamins have generally a greater potential toxicity compared with water-soluble vitamins because they are

a.  more essential to vital metabolic processes
b.  metabolically faster
c.  avidly stored by the body
d.  administered in larger doses
e.  involved in more essential metabolic pathways

**395.** In the United States, the "Recommended Daily Allowances" (RDAs) are periodically developed by the

a.  National Research Council (NRC)
b.  Food and Drug Administration (FDA)
c.  Department of Agriculture
d.  Department of Commerce
e.  Surgeon General

**396.** Which vitamin needs to be given in supplemental doses in order to prevent deficiency when a patient is given prolonged administration of isoniazid (INH)?

a.  vitamin A
b.  vitamin K
c.  vitamin C
d.  thiamine
e.  pyridoxine

**DIRECTIONS:** Each numbered question or incomplete statement below is NEGATIVELY phrased. Select the **one best** lettered response.

**397.** Which of the following is a stool softener that does NOT decrease absorption of fat-soluble vitamins?

a. mineral oil
b. castor oil
c. docusate sodium
d. phenolphthalein
e. cascara sagrada

**398.** True statements concerning sucralfate include all the following EXCEPT

a. it contains polyaluminum hydroxide
b. it maintains gel-like qualities even at acid pH
c. it binds to ulcer craters more than to normal mucosa
d. it has moderate acid-neutralizing properties
e. it reacts very little with mucin

**DIRECTIONS:** Each group of questions below consists of lettered headings followed by a set of numbered items. For each numbered item select the **one** lettered heading with which it is **most** closely associated. Each lettered heading may be used **once, more than once, or not at all.**

### Questions 399–400

Match each vitamin with the appropriate description.

a.   excess amounts should be avoided when the patient is on levodopa (L-dopa)
b.   overdosage may lead to a psychotic state
c.   improvement of vision especially in daylight might be attributable to this vitamin
d.   this vitamin is usually not included in the popular "one-a-day" vitamin preparations
e.   retinoic acid is the natural form
f.   acute intoxication with this vitamin causes hypertension, nausea and vomiting, and signs of increased cerebrospinal fluid (CSF) pressure
g.   this vitamin has hormonal functions
h.   this fat-soluble vitamin has mainly antioxidant properties
i.   in its water-soluble form, this fat-soluble vitamin is capable of producing kernicterus

**399.** Calcitriol (vitamin D metabolite—1,25-dihydroxyvitamin D)

**400.** Menadione

### Questions 401–402

For each vitamin, match the appropriate use or deficiency.

a.   large doses are used to treat hyperlipoproteinemia
b.   large doses are used to acidify urine
c.   this vitamin is used in the therapy of Wernicke's syndrome
d.   large doses are used to cure psychosis
e.   deficiency can cause angular stomatitis
f.   deficiency can cause the common cold
g.   deficiency can cause convulsions in children

**401.** Nicotinic acid (niacin)

**402.** Thiamine

(Read)

## Questions 403–404

Match the main therapeutic potential with the correct listed GI drug.

a. ranitidine
b. metronidazole
c. omeprazole
d. sucralfate
e. misoprostol
f. Ca carbonate
g. loperamide

**403.** Preferred drug therapy for Zollinger-Ellison syndrome *omeprazole*

**404.** Helpful in selected cases of diarrhea *loperamide*

## Questions 405–406

There are different mechanisms by which laxatives achieve their effects. Match the mechanism to the correct drug.

a. Mg sulfate
b. methylcellulose
c. phenolphthalein
d. castor oil
e. lactulose
f. mineral oil
g. docusate Na (dioctyl sodium sulfosuccinate)

**405.** Has a hyperosmotic mechanism different from that of saline cathartics *lactulose*

**406.** Increases colonic peristalsis and enhances fluid and electrolyte secretion into the bowel *Phenolphthalein*

## Questions 407–408

A large number of endogenous and exogenous agents act to alter the rate of secretion of acid by the parietal cell. Match the mechanism to the agent.

a. histamine
b. prostaglandin
c. gastrin
d. acetylcholine
e. aspirin
f. propantheline
g. food
h. Al hydroxide
i. bismuth subsalicylate
j. omeprazole
k. misoprostol
l. sucralfate

**407.** Lowers gastric acidity by competitive antagonism of acetylcholine *(Propantheline)*

**408.** Increases gastric acidity by preventing the action of inhibitory guanine nucleotide-binding protein (G protein) on adenylate cylase *(aspirin)*

# GASTROINTESTINAL SYSTEM AND NUTRITION

## Answers

**379. The answer is b.** (*DiPalma, 4/e, pp 199, 562. Hardman and Limbird, 9/e, p 906.*) Cimetidine reversibly inhibits cytochrome P–450. This is important in phase I biotransformation reactions and inhibits the metabolism of such drugs as warfarin, phenytoin, propranolol, metoprolol, quinidine, and theophylline. None of the other enzymes are significantly affected.

**380. The answer is d.** (*DiPalma, 4/e, p 568.*) Although Al hydroxide is generally considered to be the antacid that inhibits phosphate absorption, Ca carbonate is equally capable of this effect. This adverse effect may be hazardous in the presence of renal impairment.

**381. The answer is d.** (*DiPalma, 4/e, pp 862–863. Hardman and Limbird, 9/e, pp 907–909.*) Omeprazole inhibits $H^+/K^+/ATPase$, which effectively stops the proton pump and thus prevents the formation of gastric acid. It is the most effective agent in severe cases of ulceration and esophageal reflux.

**382. The answer is e.** (*DiPalma, 4/e, p 570. Hardman and Limbird, 9/e, p 926.*) Diphenoxylate is a piperidine opioid related to meperidine. It inhibits peristalsis and hence increases the passage time of the intestinal bolus. It is combined with atropine to discourage use as a street drug. Atropine has little effect on peristalsis. Clonidine, bismuth subsalicylate, and rehydration therapy are all useful in some types of diarrhea, but none of them inhibit peristalsis.

**383. The answer is d.** (*DiPalma, 4/e, pp 564–565. Hardman and Limbird, 9/e, p 611.*) Misoprostol is a prostaglandin E (PGE) analogue that has antisecretory and mucosal protection properties in the stomach. Experimentally it protects against mucosal damage from NSAIDs, alcohol, and other toxic agents. It will also tend to heal existing ulcers but is inferior to other agents in this regard.

**384. The answer is c.** (*DiPalma, 4/e, pp 574–575. Hardman and Limbird, 9/e, pp 932–933.*) Metoclopramide antagonizes the emetic effect of apomorphine, which is mediated by a dopamine receptor in the CNS. It also raises the lower esophageal sphincter pressure and relaxes the pyloric sphincter, which hastens gastric emptying time. This makes it useful in the therapy of reflux esophagitis.

**385. The answer is d.** (*Hardman and Limbird, 9/e, p 935 Isselbacher, 13/e, p 1530.*) Pancrelipase is an alcoholic extract of hog pancreas that contains lipase, trypsin, and amylase. It is effective in reducing the steatorrhea of pancreatic insufficiency. None of the other drugs mentioned have significant action in the digestion of fats.

**386. The answer is d.** (*Hardman and Limbird, 9/e, pp 934–935. Isselbacher, 13/e, p 1509.*) Chenodeoxycholic acid (chenodiol) and ursodiol have proved to be effective in some patients with cholesterol gallstones. Lovastatin lowers blood cholesterol levels but has no effect on gallstones. Methyl tertiary butyl ether and a new agent, monoctanoin, are infused directly into the common duct and will dissolve gallstones.

**387. The answer is b.** (*DiPalma, 4/e, p 577. Hardman and Limbird, 9/e, p 1061.*) Sulfasalazine consists of sulfapyridine with 5-aminosalicylic acid linked by an azo bond. This bond is broken by bacteria that release the salicylic acid, which is believed to be the active agent. Sulfa drugs or salicylic acid used alone is not as effective. The mechanism of action is unknown but is believed to be protective action on the mucosa by inhibition of the synthesis of prostaglandins and leukotrienes.

**388. The answer is a.** (*DiPalma, 4/e, p 573. Hardman and Limbird, 9/e, p 922.*) Lactulose is a synthetic disaccharide (galactose-fructose) that is not absorbed. In moderate doses it acts as a laxative. In higher doses it is capable of binding ammonia and other toxins that form in the intestine in severe liver deficiency and that are believed to cause the encephalopathy. Loperamide is an antidiarrheal opioid; lorazepam is a CNS depressant; loxapine is a tricyclic antipsychotic.

**389. The answer is d.** (*DiPalma, 4/e, p 566. Isselbacher, 13/e, p 1367.*) It is now recognized that infection with *Helicobacter pylori* is a major etiologic factor in peptic ulcer disease. Bismuth salts are bactericidal for many organisms but especially for spirochetes. Colloidal bismuth salts such as bismuth subsalicylate also have a coating or cytoprotective action.

**390. The answer is a.** (*DiPalma, 4/e, pp 564–565. Hardman and Limbird, 9/e, p 914.*) Misoprostol is a prostaglandin analogue of PGE with an affinity for the gastric mucosa. It stimulates the secretion of mucus and bicarbonate, enhances cell proliferation, preserves the microcirculation, and stabilizes tissue lysosomes. Misoprostol is approved by the FDA for protection against the ulcerogenic action of NSAIDs (not because it antagonizes NSAIDs).

**391. The answer is d.** (*DiPalma, 4/e, p 543. Hardman and Limbird, 9/e, p 1575.*) Isotretinoin is actually a form of high-dose vitamin A therapy. Vitamin A itself or retinol (vitamin $A_1$) could be used, but they have less advantageous pharmacokinetic properties. Antibiotics such as tetracyclines are used in acne but have little effect on the nodulocystic form.

**392. The answer is d.** (*DiPalma, 4/e, pp 562–563. Hardman and Limbird, 9/e, pp 907–909.*) The main action of omeprazole is inhibition of secretion of gastric acid. Because it is a specific inhibitor of the proton pump ($H^+/K^+/ATPase$), other actions are secondary to the marked decline of acid secretion. As a result of the reduction of gastric acidity, there is increased secretion of gastrin leading to hypergastrinemia.

**393. The answer is a.** (*DiPalma, 4/e, p 541. Hardman and Limbird, 9/e, p 1579.*) Pregnant women should not take more than a 25% increase in the normal dietary intake of vitamin A for it is definitely teratogenic, especially in the first trimester of pregnancy. Great caution is to be taken in premenopausal females in the therapy of acne and skin wrinkling in which tretinoin or isotretinoin is the therapeutic agent. None of the other vitamins is particularly teratogenic except perhaps vitamin D.

**394. The answer is c.** (*DiPalma, 4/e, pp 542, 546, 548.*) Fat-soluble vitamins, especially vitamins A and D, can be stored in massive amounts and hence have a potential for serious toxicities. Water-soluble vitamins are easily excreted by the kidney and toxic accumulation rarely occurs.

**395. The answer is a.** (*DiPalma, 4/e, p 539.*) The National Research Council has a Food and Nutrition Board, which has the function of selecting the levels of vitamins, minerals, and other substances necessary to achieve maximum nutritional health. The levels are reviewed periodically and determined by study of the nutritional needs of healthy persons. The Food and Drug Administration is responsible for labeling of nutritional products but does not determine the RDAs.

**396. The answer is e.** (*DiPalma, 4/e, p 748.*) The toxicity of INH is mainly on the peripheral and central nervous systems (PNS, CNS). This is attributable to competition of INH with pyridoxal phosphate for apotryptophanase. This results in a relative deficiency of pyridoxine, which causes peripheral neuritis, insomnia, and muscle twitching among other effects.

**397. The answer is c.** (*DiPalma, 4/e, p 573. Hardman and Limbird, 9/e, p 924.*) Dioctyl sodium sulfosuccinate (docusate) is a detergent that, when given orally, softens the stool and prevents straining. Mineral oil also softens the stool, but it tends to inhibit absorption of fat-soluble vitamins and other nutrients. Castor oil, phenolphthalein, and cascara are strong laxatives and cause watery stools.

**398. The answer is d.** (*DiPalma, 4/e, pp 565–566. Hardman and Limbird, 9/e, p 913.*) Sucralfate is a sulfated disaccharide that contains polyaluminum hydroxide. It has primarily protective properties and attaches firmly to ulcer craters. It has no significant acid-neutralizing properties.

**399–400. The answers are 399-g, 400-i.** (*DiPalma, 4/e, pp 539–556.*) Phytonadione, the fat-soluble form of vitamin K, is often not included in so-called one-a-day vitamin preparations because it is so ubiquitous in the usual diet. Only in liver disease does a deficiency of the vitamin occur.

Calcitriol (1,25-dihydroxyvitamin D) is the most active form of vitamin D. It is formed by the kidney. When the Ca blood level rises, the kidney produces 24,25-dihydroxyvitamin D, a much less active form. Vitamin D can be manufactured in the body by the action of sunlight on the skin. Its main action is to increase Ca absorption in the gut. Thus, vitamin D subserves important hormonal functions in Ca homeostasis.

Levodopa is converted to dopamine (DM) in the peripheral tissues by dopa decarboxylase, which has as a cofactor pyridoxine. Excess of this vitamin will increase this reaction, which is an undesirable effect because dopamine does not cross the blood-brain barrier where the therapeutic effect is desired.

Menadione, the water-soluble form of vitamin K, should not be given to infants because of the high incidence of hemolysis and jaundice.

α-tocopherol, or vitamin E, is relatively nontoxic and has antioxidant properties (e.g., preserving intracellular components such as ubiquinone).

**401–402. The answers are 401-a, 402-c.** (*DiPalma, 4/e, pp 539–556.*) Angular stomatitis, dermatitis, and corneal vascularization are considered classic signs of human riboflavin deficiency, although multiple B vitamins may be involved.

Nicotinic acid (niacin) in doses of 1 to 3 g a day, over 100 times the RDA, causes a significant lowering of blood cholesterol. This is not an attribute of nicotinamide. Nicotinic acid and nicotinamide are both effective in curing pellagra. Large doses of nicotinic acid have been used in attempts to cure various psychoses, but this therapy is now discredited.

Vitamin C, which is sometimes recommended in large doses for the common cold and as a cure for cancer, is actually more useful as a method of acidifying urine and increasing the excretion of such abused drugs as phencyclidine.

Pyridoxine deficiency is most common in children on infant formulas that do not contain this vitamin. Deficiency of this vitamin causes convulsions.

The classic therapy of the bizarre CNS signs and symptoms of withdrawal in severe alcoholics (Wernicke's syndrome) is intravenous administration of thiamine plus glucose infusion. Alcoholics generally have other deficiencies of vitamins, especially riboflavin and niacin.

**403–404. The answers are 403-c, 404-g.** (*DiPalma, 4/e, pp 562–563, 570. Hardman and Limbird, 9/e, pp 907–909, 926–927.*) Omeprazole, which is an inhibitor of the parietal cell $H^+/K^+/ATPase$ pump (proton pump), is the most effective means of decreasing gastric acidity. This makes it the ideal agent to treat Zollinger-Ellison syndrome, which results from increased gastric secretion due to gastrinomas.

Loperamide is an opiate that is poorly absorbed from the gastrointestinal tract but still retains the ability to inhibit peristalsis. It is useful in diarrheas that are just symptomatic and are not due to infection or organic pathology, such as inflammatory bowel disease.

**405–406. The answers are 405-e, 406-c.** (*DiPalma, 4/e, pp 572–574. Hardman and Limbird, 9/e, pp 922–923.*) Lactulose is a disaccharide that is not absorbed and thus acts as an osmotic agent in the gut. In the colon, lactulose is broken down by bacteria to lactic, formic, and acetic acids plus carbon dioxide, which tend to also increase motility.

Phenolphthalein, like anthraquinones and other irritant phenolic compounds, is a stimulant laxative. Colonic peristalsis is increased by stimulation of sensory nerve endings in the mucosa of the intestine. Phenolphthalein also enhances entrance of water and salts into the bowel.

**407–408. The answers are 407-f, 408-e.** (*DiPalma, 4/e, pp 560–561.*) Acetylcholine or vagal stimulation causes an increase in Ca in the parietal cell. This in turn stimulates protein kinase, which activates the H⁺/K⁺/ATPase pump to secrete H⁺ ions and increase acidity. Blocking the action of acetylcholine with atropine-like drugs thus results in lower gastric acidity. Propantheline is an anticholinergic that has advantages over atropine and has been widely used to treat peptic ulcer.

Prostaglandins, especially $PGE_2$ and $PGI_2$, stimulate inhibitory G protein, which controls adenylate cyclase, so as to decrease the production of cAMP and thus decrease the action of the H⁺/K⁺/ATPase pump through protein kinase. Aspirin and other NSAIDs inhibit the synthesis of prostaglandins, allowing stimulatory G protein to be activated by other mechanisms and thus allowing the parietal cell to secrete more acid. Misoprostol, a synthetic prostaglandin, is used to antagonize this action of aspirin and NSAIDs in patients who must take these drugs and who are at risk of developing peptic ulcers.

# ENDOCRINE SYSTEM

**Note: In the classification of drugs, prototype drugs are marked with an asterisk (\*)**

Anabolic Steroids
  Dromostanolone propionate
  Methandrostenolone
  Nandrolone decanoate
  Nandrolone phenpropionate
  Oxandrolone
  Oxymetholone
  Stanozolol *(Ben Johnson)*
Corticosteroids
  Beclomethasone
  Cortisone
  Dexamethasone
  Fludrocortisone
  Hydrocortisone
  Prednisone*
  Methylprednisolone
  Metyrapone ? —*2mce*
  Spironolactone
  Triamcinolone
Corticotropins
Corticotropin (Adrenocorticotropic
  Hormone [ACTH])*
  Cosyntropin
Female Sex Hormones and Oral
  Contraceptives
  Chlorotrianisene*
  Conjugated estrogens
  Danazol*
  Desogestrel
  Dienestrol

Diethylstilbestrol
Estradiol
Estrone
Estropipate
Ethinyl estradiol
Ethynodiol
Hydroxyprogesterone
Leuprolide*
Levonorgestrel (L-norgestrel)
Luteinizing hormone-releasing
  hormone (LHRH)
  (hypothalamic)
Medroxyprogesterone
Megestrol
Mestranol
Mifepristone
Norethindrone
Norethynodrel
Norgestrel
Quinestrol
Tamoxifen*
Fertility Agents
  Bromocriptine*
  Clomiphene*
  Human chorionic gonadotropin
    (hCG)
  Human menopausal
    gonadotropin (hMG)
Hyperglycemic Agents
  Diazoxide

Glucagon*

Insulins

Extended insulin zinc (Zn)
suspension

Insulin injection

Insulin Zn suspension

Isophane insulin suspension
(NPH)

70% NPH insulin suspension
+ 30% insulin injection

50% NPH insulin suspension
+ 50% insulin injection

Male Sex Hormones

Finasteride

Fluoxymesterone

Flutamide

Methyltestosterone*

Nafarelin

Testosterone*

Testosterone cypionate

Testosterone enanthate

Testosterone propionate

Spironolactone

Oral Hypoglycemic Agents

Acetohexamide

Chlorpropamide

Glipizide

Glyburide

Tolazamide

Tolbutamide*

Metformin

Parathyroid Drugs

Calcitonin*

Calcitriol (vitamin D metabolite
[active form]—1,25-dihydroxy-
vitamin D)

Calcifediol

Dihydrotachysterol

Ergocalciferol

Etidronate*

Gallium nitrate

Parathyroid hormone (PTH)

Pamidronate

Phosphates

Plicamycin (mithramycin)

Vitamin D*

Thyroid Drugs

Desiccated thyroid*

Iodide ($I^-$)

Levothyroxine ($LT_4$)

Liothyronine

Liotrix

Methimazole

Propylthiouracil (PTU)*

Protirelin

Radioactive iodine ($^{131}I$)

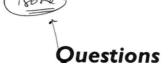
*Bone*

# Questions

**DIRECTIONS:** Each question below contains several suggested responses. Select the **one best** response to each question.

**409.** The mechanism of action of etidronate disodium is most likely related to

a. an unusual form of phosphorus (P)
b. inhibition of both normal and abnormal bone resorption
c. hyperphosphatemia
d. excretion unchanged in the urine
e. inhibition of formation of hydroxyapatite crystals

*Elevens*
*? retardation*

**410.** Glucocorticoid synthesis is under direct control of

a. the hypothalamus
b. the posterior pituitary
c. the adrenal medulla
d. corticotropin-releasing factor (CRF)
e. ACTH

**411.** A substance that enhances the probability of ovulation by blocking the inhibitory effect of estrogens and thus stimulating the release of gonadotropin from the pituitary is

a. oxymetholone
b. clomiphene
c. diethylstilbestrol
d. ethinyl estradiol
e. progesterone

**412.** A naturally occurring substance useful in treating Paget's disease of bone is

a. etidronate
b. cortisol
c. calcitonin
d. PTH
e. thyroxine ($T_4$)

*long Acting*

**413.** NPH (neural protamine Hagedorn) differs from extended insulin (Zn) suspension in which of the following actions?

a. it activates receptor tyrosine kinases
b. it causes movement of intracellular glucose transporters to the cell membrane
c. following subcutaneous injection, it reaches peak plasma concentrations by 6 to 10 h
d. it has a longer duration of action
e. it increases lipogenesis

**414.** The preferred thyroid preparation for maintenance replacement therapy is which of the following drugs?

a. desiccated thyroid
b. liothyronine
c. protirelin
d. $LT_4$
e. liotrix

**415.** A patient becomes markedly tetanic following a recent thyroidectomy. This symptom can be rapidly reversed by the administration of

a.  vitamin D
b.  calcitonin
c.  PTH
d.  plicamycin (mithramycin)
e.  calcium gluconate (CaG)

**416.** A 75-year-old diabetic female needs oral antidiabetic therapy. The patient lives alone, and you are particularly concerned about the risk of hypoglycemia. Which of the following oral antidiabetic drugs is MOST likely to cause hypoglycemia?

a.  glyburide
b.  metformin
c.  tolbutamide
d.  glipizide
e.  tolazamide

**417.** Metyrapone is useful in testing the endocrine functioning of the

a.  α cells of pancreatic islets
b.  β cells of pancreatic islets
c.  neurohypophysis
d.  pituitary-adrenal axis
e.  Leydig cells of testes

**418.** Of the following mechanisms of anti-inflammatory and immunosuppressive effects of glucocorticoids, which one is uniformly observed?

a.  increased influx of leukocytes to the site of inflammation
b.  reduced formation of lipocortins
c.  reduced capillary permeability and edema at the inflammatory site
d.  increased prostaglandin formation
e.  enhanced formation of interleukins (IL-1, IL-2)

**419.** Bromocriptine is used to treat some cases of amenorrhea because it

a.  stimulates release of gonadotropin-releasing hormone (GnRH)
b.  stimulates the ovary directly
c.  is an estrogen antagonist that enhances gonadotropin release
d.  inhibits prolactin release
e.  increases the synthesis of follicle-stimulating hormone (FSH)

**420.** Tamoxifen is used to treat some breast cancers because of its ability to

a.  utilize its androgenic properties in retarding tumor growth
b.  prevent estrogen synthesis by the ovary
c.  enhance glucocorticoid treatment
d.  act as an estrogen antagonist
e.  act as a potent progestin

**421.** Concern is raised in an 86-year-old male with noninsulin-dependent diabetes mellitus (NIDDM), or type II diabetes, about the possibility of hypoglycemia when considering the use of an oral hypoglycemic agent. Which of the following antidiabetic drugs is LEAST likely to cause hypoglycemia?

a. metformin
b. chlorpropamide
c. insulin
d. glipizide

**422.** The most dangerous adverse reaction to the administration of methimazole is

a. hypothyroidism
b. arthralgia
c. jaundice
d. agranulocytosis
e. renal toxicity

**423.** The initial and crucial event that enables tolbutamide to cause the pancreatic β cells to release insulin is

a. increased potassium (K) efflux
b. binding to receptors on the adenosine triphosphate (ATP)-sensitive K⁺ channels
c. closing of voltage-dependent Ca channels
d. decreased phosphorylation reactions
e. hyperpolarization

**424.** The treatment of myxedema coma can include which of the following agents?

a. thyroglobulin
b. $LT_4$
c. lithium
d. PTU
e. protirelin

**425.** The "minipill" containing only a progestin, rather than a combination estrogen-progestin oral contraceptive, was developed because progestin alone

a. results in less depression and cholestatic jaundice
b. is a more effective contraceptive agent than the two combined
c. results in a more regular menstrual cycle
d. is thought to be less likely to induce endometriosis
e. is thought to be less likely to induce cardiovascular disorders

**426.** PTH has which one of the following effects?

a. increased mobilization of Ca from bone
b. decreased active absorption of Ca from the small intestine
c. decreased renal tubular reabsorption of Ca
d. decreased resorption of phosphate from bone
e. decreased excretion of phosphate

**DIRECTIONS:** Each numbered question or incomplete statement below is NEGATIVELY phrased. Select the **one best** lettered response.

**427.** The general structure for thyroid hormones is shown below. In order for this structure to acquire significant hormone activity, all the following modifications must take place EXCEPT that

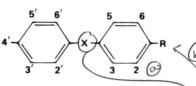

a. the connection between the two aromatic rings should be by ether, thioether, or methylene linkage
b. the R side chain on carbon 1 should be aliphatic and contain a carboxyl group
c. halogenation or methylation is necessary at positions 3 and 5
d. a hydroxyl group should be on position 39
e. position 49 should have a hydroxyl group or a group capable of being metabolically converted to hydroxyl

**428.** Drugs that bind to receptors in the plasma membrane and enhance levels of cyclic 3′,5′-adenosine monophosphate (cyclic AMP [cAMP]) include all the following EXCEPT

a. ACTH
b. calcitonin
c. isoproterenol
d. hydrocortisone
e. glucagon

**429.** True statements about testosterone include all the following EXCEPT

a. it is biotransformed primarily in the liver
b. it enhances the excretion of sodium (Na) and water
c. it has a stimulatory effect on hematopoietic cells
d. it attaches to a receptor on the X chromosome
e. it is converted to an active metabolite, dihydrotestosterone (DHT)

**430.** Glucocorticoids are powerful anti-inflammatory agents. Which of the following is NOT an anti-inflammatory mechanism of action of glucocorticoids?

a. decreased secretion of proteolytic enzymes
b. reduction in release of cytokines, such as IL-1 and IL-2
c. decreased number of circulating neutrophils
d. impairment of prostaglandin and leukotriene synthesis

**431.** Inhibition of the peripheral conversion of thyroxine ($T_4$) to triiodothyronine ($T_3$) by the liver and kidney is caused by all the following drugs EXCEPT

a.  propranolol
b.  amiodarone
c.  hydrocortisone
d.  methimazole  *(coupling)*
e.  PTU

**432.** All the following are steroid compounds EXCEPT

a.  mestranol
b.  clomiphene
c.  ethynodiol diacetate
d.  norethindrone
e.  beclomethasone

**433.** Abuse of anabolic steroids by athletes can result in all the following EXCEPT

a.  retention of fluid
b.  feminization in males
c.  decreased spermatogenesis
d.  depression
e.  anorexia

**434.** Drugs that increase the need for insulin include all the following EXCEPT

a.  epinephrine
b.  hydrocortisone
c.  chlorthalidone
d.  dexamethasone
e.  ethanol (acute ingestion)

**435.** Drugs that enter the cytoplasm of a cell and then bind to a specific receptor include all the following EXCEPT

a.  trihexyphenidyl
b.  triamcinolone
c.  mestranol
d.  fludrocortisone
e.  calcitriol

*steroid moiety*

**436.** Accurate statements about calcitriol include all the following EXCEPT

a.  it is formed in the kidney from calcifediol by hydroxylation
b.  it may cause arrhythmias in digitalized patients
c.  it has a rapid onset of action
d.  it is 25-$OH_3$-vitamin $D_3$
e.  it enhances intestinal absorption of Ca

**437.** Adverse reactions to administration of chlorpropamide include all the following EXCEPT

a.  water retention
b.  increased tolerance to ethanol
c.  hypoglycemia
d.  hyponatremia
e.  exacerbation of peptic ulcers

**438.** True statements about danazol include all the following EXCEPT

a.  it is a testosterone derivative
b.  it can cause edema
c.  it can cause gynecomastia
d.  it can decrease high-density lipoprotein (HDL) cholesterol
e.  it is indicated in endometriosis

**439.** Hypervitaminosis D produces all the following effects EXCEPT

a.   nephrocalcinosis
b.   polyuria
c.   osteoporosis
d.   polydipsia
e.   mild alkalosis

**440.** Adverse reactions associated with methylprednisolone include all the following EXCEPT

a.   osteoporosis
b.   peptic ulceration
c.   increased susceptibility to infection
d.   hypoglycemia
e.   edema

**441.** Glyburide has all the following attributes EXCEPT

a.   it is mildly diuretic
b.   it promotes the release of insulin
c.   it is a second-generation oral hypo-glycemic agent
d.   its duration of action is 12 to 24 h and the drug may be given once a day
e.   it may decrease tolerance to ethanol

**442.** All the following drugs can cause hyperglycemia and hypo-kalemia EXCEPT

a.   hydrocortisone
b.   chlorpropamide
c.   hydrochlorothiazide
d.   bumetanide
e.   prednisone

**443.** All the following compounds reduce the effectiveness of chlor-propamide EXCEPT

a.   phenobarbital
b.   chlorothiazide
c.   furosemide
d.   diazoxide
e.   salicylates

**DIRECTIONS:** Each group of questions below consists of lettered headings followed by a set of numbered items. For each numbered item select the **one** lettered heading with which it is **most** closely associated. Each lettered heading may be used **once, more than once, or not at all.**

## Questions 444–446

Match each clinical use or entity below with the most appropriate drug.

a.   mifepristone
b.   spironolactone
c.   aminoglutethimide
d.   leuprolide
e.   fludrocortisone

**444.** An abortifacient

**445.** Mineralocorticoid replacement therapy in primary adrenal insufficiency

**446.** Advanced prostate cancer

## Questions 447–449

For each inhibitory effect on the synthesis of thyroid hormone listed below, select the agent that causes it.

a.   Na thiocyanate
b.   methimazole
c.   triiodothyronine
d.   $^{131}$I
e.   I$^-$

**447.** Inhibits, by acting as a competitor, the accumulation of I$^-$ in thyroid follicular cells

**448.** Inhibits the peroxidase-catalyzed oxidation of I$^-$ and thus interferes with the incorporation of I$^-$ into an organic structure

**449.** Inhibits the peroxidase-catalyzed coupling of iodotyrosines to form iodothyronines

**450.** A 53-year-old female with NIDDM is started on a sulfonylurea. Which of the following is one mechanism of action of sulfonylureas?

a.   they increase insulin synthesis
b.   they release preformed insulin
c.   they directly promote glucose uptake by muscle, liver, and adipose tissue

**451.** A 29-year-old female who takes LT$_4$ following her thyroidectomy becomes pregnant. If the dosage is not changed, she will become:

a.   hyperthyroid
b.   euthyroid
c.   hypothyroid

**452.** A 37-year-old female with Graves' disease who requires antithyroid therapy becomes pregnant. Which antithyroid drug is safest?

a.   potassium iodide (KI)
b.   methimazole
c.   PTU
d.   potassium perchlorate (KClO$_4$)

## Questions 453–455

Match each statement with the correct drug.

a. aldosterone
b. clomiphene
c. diazoxide
d. fludrocortisone
e. NPH
f. methimazole
g. Ethinyl estradiol
h. norethindrone
i. norethynodrel
j. PTU
k. salicylates
l. spironolactone
m. tamoxifen
n. triamcinolone

**453.** This drug promotes the synthesis of factors II, VII, IX, and X and may interfere with the effect of warfarin or may result in thromboembolic phenomena *ethyl estradiol*

**454.** The therapeutic effect of this drug is reduced by glucocorticoids, dextrothyroxine, epinephrine, hydrochlorothiazide, and LT$_4$. *(NPH)*

**455.** This drug reduces the growth of facial hair in idiopathic hirsutism or hirsutism secondary to androgen excess *spironolactone*

**456.** A 36-year-old male has had a thyroidectomy and now requires maintenance therapy. Which of the following is the drug of choice?

a. KI
b. PTU
c. triiodothyronine
d. ipodate
e. T$_4$

**457.** A 27-year-old female is diagnosed with hypercortisolism. To determine whether cortisol production is independent of the pituitary gland, you decide to suppress ACTH production by giving a high-potency glucocorticoid. Which glucocorticoid is the best for this indication?

a. triamcinolone
b. prednisone
c. hydrocortisone
d. dexamethasone
e. methylprednisolone

**458.** A 22-year-old female carrying a preterm pregnancy (33 weeks) is in labor. Which of the following drugs can be given to the mother to promote fetal lung maturity?

a. betamethasone
b. fludrocortisone
c. metyrapone
d. spironolactone
e. triamcinolone

*Beta > Dexa.*

**459.** A 48-year-old female is diagnosed with small cell lung carcinoma with ectopic production of ACTH. An adrenocortical antagonist (drug X) is given, and cortisol levels decrease significantly. Following treatment, the patient complains of excess hair growth and swelling of the legs. What is drug X?

a. metyrapone
b. aminoglutethimide
c. spironolactone
d. ketoconazole

**460.** A 22-year-old male with a five-year history of bronchial asthma has developed increased frequency and severity of acute asthmatic attacks. A low dose of which inhaled steroid is added to his treatment regimen?

a. prednisolone
b. amcinonide
c. beclomethasone
d. cortisone
e. fluocinolone

**461.** A 76-year-old male complains of progressive difficulty starting his stream on urinating and getting up at least once each night to urinate. Rectal examination reveals a generally enlarged, smooth-surfaced prostate. Prostatic serum antigen is 0.2 nanograms per milliliter (ng/mL). Finasteride therapy is begun and results in improved urine flow and decreased prostate size. What is this drug's mechanism of action?

a. inhibition of the testosterone receptor
b. inhibition of steroid 5α-reductase
c. inhibition of testosterone synthesis
d. inhibition of the GnRH receptor

**Questions 462–464**

For each patient, select the drug that was given:

a. spironolactone
b. furosemide
c. clomiphene
d. propranolol
e. medroxyprogesterone
f. chlorpropamide
g. plicamycin (mithramycin)
h. phentolamine

**462.** A 25-year-old female complains of increasing anxiety and "restlessness." Physical examination reveals tachycardia and tremors. Palpation of the neck reveals a 3 cm nodule on her thyroid gland. While awaiting laboratory confirmation of the diagnosis, she is given a drug that diminishes her tachycardia and tremors.

**463.** A 48-year-old male with a three-year history of carcinoma of the colon complains of intense pain in his hips. X-rays suggest tumor infiltrates. His serum Ca is 11.5 milliequivalents per liter (mEq/L). A therapeutic regimen is begun that contains a drug that lowers the serum Ca to 8.9 mEq/L.

**464.** A 50-year-old female had a radical mastectomy three years ago for hormone-dependent breast adenocarcinoma. She is now complaining of shortness of breath, and chest X-ray shows diffuse lung metastases. As part of her therapeutic regimen, she is given intramuscular (IM) HRT.

# ENDOCRINE SYSTEM

## Answers

**409. The answer is e.** (*DiPalma, 4/e, pp 594–595. Hardman and Limbird, 9/e, pp 1537–1538.*) Etidronate is used in the treatment of Paget's disease of bone. The compound is classified as a diphosphonate. It can be administered orally or by injection. The drug affects both normal and abnormal bone resorption and appears to reduce the activity of osteoclasts and osteoblasts. It inhibits the formation, growth, and dissolution of hydroxyapatite crystals, which is probably its main mechanism of action. There occurs a significant reduction in serum Ca following several days of intravenous therapy with etidronate. The drug has a half-life of about 6 h and is excreted unchanged in the urine. Etidronate has also been used to treat patients with hypercalcemia that may be associated with various neoplastic diseases.

**410. The answer is e.** (*DiPalma, 4/e, pp 638–639. Hardman and Limbird, 9/e, pp 1461–1464.*) Glucocorticoid synthesis is under the control of ACTH. In response to the release of CRF, corticotropin is elaborated from the anterior pituitary gland. It is a polypeptide of 39 amino acids. In the body, cortisol (hydrocortisone) exerts a negative feedback mechanism to suppress the release of corticotropin. Corticotropin affects lipid metabolism by producing a stimulatory effect on lipolysis, which results in an elevated plasma concentration of free fatty acids. The drug is used in the diagnosis of adrenal insufficiency (e.g., primary adrenal insufficiency). When it is given intravenously, its half-life is short, lasting about 15 min. A synthetic form of corticotropin is cosyntropin, which contains only the first 24 amino acids of the peptide.

**411. The answer is b.** (*DiPalma, 4/e, pp 619–620. Hardman and Limbird, 9/e, pp 1424–1426.*) Clomiphene is an effective fertility drug that can lead to multiple pregnancies. Clomiphene has been termed an antiestrogen because its stimulant effect on the secretion of pituitary gonadotropins is thought to be the consequence of its blocking the inhibitory effect of estrogens on gonadotropin secretion. Side effects of this drug can include alopecia, breast engorgement, and hot flashes. Oxymetholone is an orally effective anabolic steroid.

**412. The answer is c.** *(DiPalma, 4/e, pp 591–595. Hardman and Limbird, 9/e, pp 1536–1537.)* Calcitonin is useful in the therapy of Paget's disease of bone (osteitis deformans). Calcitonin therapy reduces urinary hydroxyproline excretion and serum alkaline phosphatase activity and provides some symptomatic relief. Presumably these effects result from the ability of calcitonin to inhibit bone resorption. Side effects of long-term therapy with this hormone can include nausea, edema of the hands, and urticaria. The appearance of neutralizing antibodies may explain the development of resistance to treatment. Etidronate is a synthetic drug that is useful in Paget's disease. The compound is orally effective and lacks the antigenicity associated with calcitonin.

**413. The answer is d.** *(DiPalma, 4/e, pp 37–39, 599–602. Hardman and Limbird, 9/e, pp 1491–1493, 1500–1501.)* NPH (neutral protamine Hagedorn) is obtained from animal sources (beef and pork) and by recombinant deoxyribonucleic acid (DNA) techniques to yield human insulin. Protamine and Zn are contained in NPH insulin. Following subcutaneous injection it has a maximum effect of 8 to 10 h that corresponds to its peak plasma concentrations (6 to 10 h). The duration of action is 18 to 26 h, which is shorter than the duration of action of extended insulin Zn suspension. On the cellular membrane, insulin binds to receptor tyrosine kinases. The activation of these receptor tyrosine kinases leads to phosphorylation reactions and the movement of glucose transporters from the intracellular space to the membranes, where they facilitate the entrance of glucose into the cell. Insulin lowers plasma glucose levels, increases lipogenesis, decreases lipolysis and ketogenesis, and enhances the uptake of amino acids to promote protein synthesis and growth of tissues.

**414. The answer is d.** *(AMA Drug Evaluations Annual, 1993, pp 991–993. DiPalma, 4/e, pp 587–589.)* The drug of choice for maintenance replacement therapy of hypothyroidism is $LT_4$. Monitoring of plasma blood levels of $T_3$ and $T_4$ from the administration of $LT_4$ causes less difficulty than the monitoring of plasma hormone levels from liothyronine ($T_3$) because considerable fluctuation can occur with plasma concentrations of $T_3$. In addition $T_3$ has a shorter half-life. Liotrix is a mixture of $T_4$ and $T_3$ in a ratio of 4:1 that is designed to resemble the physiologic secretion of the thyroid gland.

When liotrix is administered, the $T_4$ component is converted to $T_3$ in the body, and $T_3$, therefore, is actually not needed. It does not appear that liotrix provides any therapeutic advantage over $LT_4$ by itself for the usual treatment of hypothyroidism. The treatment of hypothyroidism with desiccated thyroid is obsolete. Protirelin, a synthetic tripeptide, is chemically identical to thyrotropin-releasing hormone (TRH). This compound is used for the diagnosis of mild cases of hypothyroidism or hyperthyroidism.

**415. The answer is e.** (*DiPalma, 4/e, pp 591–594. Hardman and Limbird, 9/e, p 1523.*) Administration of intravenous CaG would immediately correct the tetany that might occur in a patient in whom a thyroidectomy was recently performed. Parathyroid hormone would act more slowly but could be given for its future stabilizing effect. Long-term control of a patient after a thyroidectomy can be obtained with vitamin D and dietary therapy. Calcitonin is a hypocalcemic antagonist of parathyroid hormone. Plicamycin (mithramycin) is used to treat Paget's disease and hypercalcemia. The dose employed is about one-tenth the amount used for plicamycin's cytotoxic action.

**416. The answer is a.** (*Hardman and Limbird, 9/e, p 1509. Katzung, 7/e, pp 698–699.*) Glyburide is a potent second-generation sulfonylurea. Compared with other oral hypoglycemics, it has a relatively long duration of action and high efficacy; therefore, it has a strong tendency to cause hypoglycemia and should be avoided in elderly patients, in whom this can be difficult to diagnose and particularly dangerous.

**417. The answer is d.** (*DiPalma, 4/e, p 647. Hardman and Limbird, 9/e, p 1482–1488.*) Metyrapone, because it decreases serum levels of cortisol by inhibiting the $11\beta$-hydroxylation of steroids in the adrenal, can be used to assess the function of the pituitary-adrenal axis. When metyrapone is administered orally or intravenously to normal persons, the adenohypophysis will secrete an increased amount of ACTH. This will cause a normal adrenal gland to synthesize increased amounts of 17-hydroxylated steroids that can be measured in the urine. However, patients who have disease of the hypothalamico-pituitary complex are not able to respond to administration of metyrapone by producing increased amounts of ACTH; consequently, no increased levels of 17-hydroxylated steroids would be detected in the urine. Before administering the drug, the ability of the adrenal gland to respond to ACTH must be tested.

**418. The answer is c.** (*DiPalma, 4/e, pp 640–643. Hardman and Limbird, 9/e, pp 1470–1472.*) Glucocorticoid compounds are used in therapy because of their anti-inflammatory and immunosuppressive properties. These steroids prevent the movement of neutrophils from the blood to the site of inflammation and cause a redistribution of leukocytes, which also reduces their influx to the site of inflammation. Glucocorticoids decrease the synthesis of prostaglandins by causing the production of lipocortin, which inhibits the enzyme phospholipase $A_2$. With the inhibition of phospholipase $A_2$, arachidonic acid is not released and as a consequence the synthesis of the prostaglandins is decreased or prevented. Glucocorticoids decrease capillary permeability and edema in the site of inflammation by decreasing vasodilation. These drugs inhibit the effects of IL-1, IL-2, tumor necrosis factor (TNF), macrophage migration inhibitory factor (MIF), and other components of the inflammatory and immune responses.

**419. The answer is d.** (*DiPalma, 4/e, p 628. Hardman and Limbird, 9/e, pp 1371–1372.*) High prolactin levels in the serum result in amenorrhea, for reasons that are not known. Bromocriptine inhibits prolactin secretion through its dopaminergic action. This compound, a semisynthetic ergot derivative, appears to be a dopamine receptor agonist. It is administered orally to the patient, and in most cases menses occurs after a month of therapy.

**420. The answer is d.** (*DiPalma, 4/e, p 619. Hardman and Limbird, 9/e, pp 1275–1276.*) Tamoxifen is an estrogen antagonist used in the treatment of breast cancer. Postmenopausal women with metastases to soft tissue and whose tumors contain an estrogen receptor are more likely to respond to this agent. Little benefit is derived from tamoxifen if the tumor does not have estrogen receptors.

**421. The answer is a.** (*Hardman and Limbird, 9/e, p 1510.*) Although the mechanism of action of metformin and other biguanides is unclear, biguanides virtually never cause hypoglycemia. They operate independently of pancreatic β cells, but are not useful in insulin-dependent diabetes mellitus (IDDM). Some possible mechanisms of action are direct stimulation of glycolysis in peripheral tissues, increased sensitivity to insulin, and reduction of glucagon levels.

**422. The answer is d.** (*DiPalma, 4/e, p 588. Hardman and Limbird, 9/e, pp 1398–1400.*) Methimazole is classified as a thioamide and is used in the treatment of hyperthyroidism. It prevents the organification of I⁻ by blocking the oxidation of I⁻ to active I and also inhibits coupling of iodotyrosines. Excessive treatment with this drug may induce hypothyroidism. Some other adverse reactions reported for methimazole include skin rash, fever, jaundice, nephritis, arthralgia, and edema. Agranulocytosis, which is a very serious reaction and may be fatal, is the most dangerous adverse reaction, but it occurs in less than 1% of patients. Patients should be carefully monitored while they are taking this medication because agranulocytosis appears without warning.

**423. The answer is b.** *(DiPalma, 4/e, pp 598–599. Hardman and Limbird, 9/e, pp 1507–1510.)* Tolbutamide is an oral hypoglycemic agent that is classified as a sulfonylurea derivative. This compound is used in the treatment of NIDDM. For hypoglycemic action, tolbutamide needs functional β cells in the pancreas, since it is ineffective in depancreatized or severely insulin-deficient patients. Sulfonylurea compounds stimulate the release of insulin from the pancreas by a proposed mechanism of action involving the initial binding of the drug to a receptor on the ATP-sensitive K channels in the cell. As a consequence of this drug-receptor interaction, there is an inhibition of K efflux from the cell, which then produces depolarization of the membrane. The depolarization of the membrane opens voltage-dependent Ca channels to allow the entrance of Ca into the cell. The increased Ca concentration stimulates phosphorylation reactions, followed by the process of exocytosis, which causes the release of insulin from the β cells. Other drugs, such as diazoxide and epinephrine, reduce insulin secretion by causing hyperpolarization of the cell, decreasing Ca ion influx, and thereby preventing the process of exocytosis for the release of insulin.

**424. The answer is b.** *(AMA Drug Evaluations Annual, 1993, p 988. DiPalma, 4/e, pp 587–589.)* Myxedema coma is a medical emergency and should be treated as soon as the diagnosis is established. Treatment involves the use of several drugs to correct this condition. It appears that the selection of either LT₄, liothyronine, or liotrix is appropriate. LT₄, however, is the drug of choice. Supportive treatment of symptoms is also indicated. Maintenance of respiration and administration of fluids and electrolytes, along with glucose if hypoglycemia is diagnosed, should be provided. Since adrenal insufficiency may be present, administration of glucocorticoids is initially recommended. Thyroglobulin, a protein of high molecular weight, is a component of the thyroid gland. Although preparations are available, this drug is not indicated in myxedema coma. Protirelin is a synthetic thyrotropin-stimulating hormone used in the diagnosis of thyroid function. Although lithium was once tested as a drug to treat hyperthyroidism because it induced hypothyroidism, lithium has no place in the therapy of hyperthyroidism. In addition, PTU is an antithyroid drug used in the management of hyperthyroidism.

**425. The answer is e.** (*DiPalma, 4/e, pp 621–627. Hardman and Limbird, 9/e, pp 1432, 1434.*) The combination of estrogen and progestin is a more effective means of contraception than is progestin alone. Menstruation will occur with progestin alone, but it may be irregular. Estrogen is thought to cause the increased incidence of thrombophlebitis and cerebral and coronary thrombosis that is found in women taking combined oral contraceptives.

**426. The answer is a.** (*DiPalma, 4/e, pp 590–594. Hardman and Limbird, 9/e, pp 1525–1528.*) PTH is synthesized by and released from the parathyroid gland; increased synthesis of PTH is a response to low serum Ca concentrations. Resorption and mobilization of Ca and phosphate from bone are increased in response to elevated PTH concentrations. Replacement of body stores of Ca is enhanced by the capacity of PTH to promote increased absorption of Ca by the small intestine in concert with vitamin D, which is the primary factor that enhances intestinal Ca absorption. PTH also causes an increased renal tubular reabsorption of Ca and excretion of phosphate. As a consequence of these effects, the extracellular Ca concentration becomes elevated.

**427. The answer is d.** (*DiPalma, 4/e, pp 583–584. Hardman and Limbird, 9/e, p 1384.*) According to extensive research on the relationship between structure and activity of thyronine derivatives, significant thyroid hormone activity would be characteristic of the structure below.

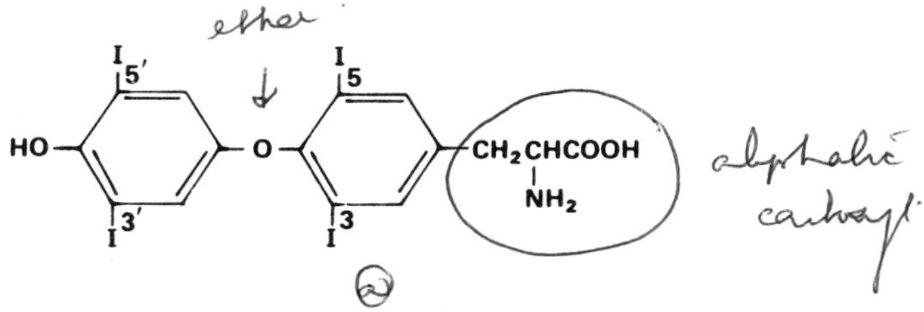

This structure is thyroxine, in which the R side chain is L-alanine, the aromatic rings are connected by an ether linkage, halogenation by I occurs on positions 3,5 and 3′,5′, and a hydroxyl group is attached to carbon 4′.

Activity can be increased fourfold upon removing I from the 5′ position because 3′-monosubstituted compounds have more activity than 3′,5′-disubstituted derivatives of thyronine.

**428. The answer is d.** (*DiPalma, 4/e, pp 34–37, 640.*) Cyclic AMP (cAMP) is an intracellular second messenger that is involved in the mechanism of action associated with adrenocorticotropic hormone, calcitonin, isoproterenol, and glucagon. These agents complex with a plasma membrane receptor that brings about the binding of guanosine triphosphate (GTP) to the coupling protein and the activation of adenylate cyclase. Adenylate cyclase catalyzes the formation of cAMP from ATP. In the cytoplasm cAMP activates cAMP-dependent protein kinase, which participates in the phosphorylation of specific substrate proteins (e.g., enzymes). The phosphorylated protein eventually induces the particular response on the target cell that is associated with the administered drug. The cellular mechanism of action of hydrocortisone, a glucocorticoid, is also related to proteins but not by the enhancement of cAMP production. Hydrocortisone is transported by simple diffusion across the membrane of the cell into the cytoplasm and binds to a specific receptor. The steroid-receptor complex is activated and enters the nucleus, where it regulates transcription of specific gene sequences into ribonucleic acid (RNA). Eventually messenger RNA (mRNA) is translated to form specific proteins in the cytoplasm that are involved in the steroid-induced cellular response.

**429. The answer is b.** (*DiPalma, 4/e, pp 630–632, 634. Hardman and Limbird, 9/e, pp 1450–1453.*) In many tissues testosterone is transformed into DHT by 5α-reductase. This active metabolite is more potent than testosterone and appears to be responsible for the androgenic effects in the body. The affinity of dihydrotestosterone is 10 times that of testosterone for the androgen-receptor gene that is located on the X chromosome. The compound testosterone is eliminated from the body through biotransformation in the liver and excretion of its metabolites, 17-ketosteroids, in the urine. Adverse reactions of testosterone and its various derivatives include virilism in prepubertal males and masculinization in females. Some other untoward effects are liver dysfunction, hypercalcemia, and retention of Na and water. Therapeutic uses of androgenic compounds are in the area of male hypogonadism, certain types of breast carcinomas, and anemia. Androgens are used in some forms of anemia because they cause the release of erythropoietin-stimulating factor, which increases production of red blood cells.

**430. The answer is c.** (*Hardman and Limbird 9/e, p 1471. Katzung, 7/e, p 639.*) Glucocorticoids actually increase the number of circulating neutrophils as inhibition of margination and migration occurs. Paradoxically, this is an anti-inflammatory effect as neutrophils had not been reaching the sites where they were needed. All of the other choices are anti-inflammatory mechanisms of glucocorticoid action.

**431. The answer is d.** (*AMA Drug Evaluations Annual, 1993, pp 983–984, 992–993. DiPalma, 4/e, pp 583–587.*) $T_3$ and $T_4$ are released from the thyroid gland and enter the circulation. $T_4$ is converted to $T_3$, which is more potent in activity, by the liver and kidney. This conversion reaction is inhibited by propranolol, amiodarone, hydrocortisone, and PTU. Although methimazole and PTU inhibit the enzymatic oxidation of $I^-$ ion to active I, which is their principal mechanism as antithyroid drugs, only PTU can block the peripheral conversion of $T_4$ to $T_3$. Propranolol and hydrocortisone are used in the treatment of certain cases of hyperthyroidism, and whether the reduction in the conversion of $T_4$ to $T_3$ plays a significant role in their mechanism of action is not fully known. The compound amiodarone is an antiarrhythmic drug that is similar in chemical structure to thyroxine.

**432. The answer is b.** (*DiPalma, 4/e, pp 615, 619–620. Hardman and Limbird, 9/e, p 1424.*) All the compounds listed in the question are steroids with the exception of clomiphene, an estrogen analogue that lacks the essential feature of a steroid, a hydrogenated cyclopentenophenanthrene-ring system. Clomid is a derivative of the weakly estrogenic compound chlorotrianisene. The compound has high antiestrogenic activity that inhibits estrogenic feedback repression of gonadotropic secretion. Clomid is an effective fertility-inducing drug.

**433. The answer is e.** (*DiPalma, 4/e, p 635. Hardman and Limbird, 9/e, pp 1451–1452.*) The use of anabolic steroids by athletes has become quite alarming in recent years. These steroids, which have androgenic and anabolic effects, are used to improve the performance of athletes in various competitive sports. Continued use of anabolic steroids induces mood changes as well as mental disorders from depression to psychosis. The androgenic properties of these drugs cause masculinization in females and may produce feminization in males. This latter effect is due to increased formation of estrogens. In addition, these steroids decrease production of endogenous testosterone by the testes and may cause a reduction in spermatogenesis. The weight gain that occurs with the administration of anabolic steroids may be due to fluid retention and an improved appetite rather than actual tissue growth. These drugs cause liver damage and increase the risk of cardiovascular diseases.

**434. The answer is e.** (*DiPalma, 4/e, pp 257, 457–460, 644.*) The regulation of levels of blood glucose by insulin and the general effectiveness of insulin are altered with the coadministration of other drugs. Epinephrine enhances glycogenolysis and thereby elevates glucose in the plasma. Glucocorticoids (e.g., hydrocortisone and dexamethasone) stimulate gluconeogenesis, reduce the peripheral utilization of glucose, and decrease the sensitivity of tissues to insulin. Chlorthalidone, a thiazide-related diuretic, may induce hyperglycemia by inhibition of the release of insulin and decrease use of glucose by peripheral tissues. In the presence of ethanol, the effect of insulin is enhanced. When ethanol is acutely ingested in sufficient quantities, the drug causes an alteration in carbohydrate metabolism that results in hypoglycemia. The exact mechanism of the hypoglycemic effect of ethanol is not known.

**435. The answer is a.** (*DiPalma, 4/e, pp 39–40, 316, 616, 630, 640.*) A variety of drugs that resemble steroid hormones in their structure can traverse cellular membranes and bind to specific cytoplasmic receptors. Triamcinolone (a glucocorticoid), fludrocortisone (a mineralocorticoid), mestranol (a sex steroid), and calcitriol (a vitamin D metabolite) all bind reversibly to the cytoplasmic receptor, which then undergoes an irreversible activation step. Next, the steroid-receptor complex enters the nucleus of the cell and regulates transcription of specific genes into RNA. Eventually mRNA is formed and causes the synthesis of specific proteins that mediate the steroid response. The response occurs 30 min to several hours following administration of the drug, since a period of time is required for formation of new proteins in the cell. Trihexyphenidyl is a synthetic anticholinergic drug that binds to muscarinic receptors associated with the cell membrane. This drug is used in the treatment of parkinsonism.

**436. The answer is d.** (*AMA Drug Evaluations Annual, 1993, p 2204. DiPalma, 4/e, pp 592–594.*) Vitamin $D_3$ is hydroxylated to 25–$OHD_3$ (calcifediol). Calcifediol is then hydroxylated in the kidney to the most active form of vitamin D, which is 1,25-dihydroxyvitamin D (calcitriol). Calcitriol has a rapid onset of action and a short half-life. The administration of calcitriol causes the elevation of serum Ca levels by enhancing the intestinal absorption of Ca. Calcitriol is indicated in vitamin D deficiency, particularly in patients with chronic renal failure or renal tubular disease, hypoparathyroidism, osteomalacia, and rickets. In patients who are treated with a digitalis preparation, it is possible for a drug interaction to occur between digitalis and drugs, such as calcitriol, that can induce hypercalcemia. Elevation of serum Ca by calcitriol in the presence of digitalis glycosides can precipitate arrhythmias.

**437. The answer is b.** (*AMA Drug Evaluations Annual, 1993, pp 1028–1032. DiPalma, 4/e, pp 604–608.*) The oral hypoglycemic agent chlorpropamide is a sulfonylurea compound. The drug is used to treat selected patients with non-insulin-dependent diabetes mellitus (NIDDM). Chlorpropamide has a duration of action of 1 to 3 days. The adverse reaction of hypoglycemia appears to be more common with chlorpropamide than with the other sulfonylurea oral hypoglycemic agents. In addition, water retention and hyponatremia can be caused by chlorpropamide. This adverse reaction is due to an interaction between antidiuretic hormone (ADH) and chlorpropamide. In the collecting duct region of the nephron, chlorpropamide may enhance the effect of antidiuretic hormone and facilitate its release from the posterior pituitary gland. It is reported that chlorpropamide decreases the tolerance to ethanol—an interaction exhibited by flushing of the skin, particularly in the facial area. This disulfiram-like effect is attributed to the inhibition of the oxidation of acetaldehyde that is formed from the biotransformation of ethanol.

**438. The answer is c.** (*AMA Drug Evaluations Annual, 1993, pp 1076, 1091. DiPalma, 4/e, pp 620, 634.*) Danazol is a 17α-ethinyl testosterone derivative used to treat endometriosis. It appears to be more effective than an estrogen-progestin combination. Since danazol is an androgen derivative, some of the adverse reactions include liver dysfunction, virilism (acne, hirsutism, oily skin, reduced breast size), and reduction in high-density lipoprotein (HDL) cholesterol levels. Other adverse reactions reported for danazol are amenorrhea, weight gain, sweating, vasomotor flushing, and edema. When danazol therapy for endometriosis was compared with the estrogen-progestin regimen, few women discontinued the treatment with danazol because of adverse reactions.

**439. The answer is e.** (*DiPalma, 4/e, pp 592–594. Hardman and Limbird, 9/e, p 1533.*) Enthusiastic overmedication with vitamin D may lead to a toxic syndrome called hypervitaminosis D. The initial symptoms can include weakness, nausea, weight loss, anemia, and mild acidosis. As the excessive doses are continued, signs of nephrotoxicity are manifested, such as polyuria, polydipsia, azotemia, and eventually nephrocalcinosis. In adults osteoporosis can occur. Also there is CNS impairment, which can result in mental retardation and convulsions.

**440. The answer is d.** (*DiPalma, 4/e, pp 644–648. Hardman and Limbird, 9/e, pp 1475–1476.*) The incidence of adverse reactions with administration of methylprednisolone is related to dosage and duration. Psychoses, peptic ulceration with or without hemorrhage, increased susceptibility to infection, edema, osteoporosis, myopathy, and hypokalemic alkalosis can occur. Other adverse reactions include cataracts, hyperglycemia, arrest of growth in children, and iatrogenic Cushing's syndrome. The glucocorticoids are very effective drugs, but they can be very dangerous if not properly administered to a patient.

**441. The answer is e.** (*AMA Drug Evaluations Annual, 1993, pp 1028–1033. DiPalma, 4/e, pp 604–607.*) Glyburide is classified as a second-generation oral hypoglycemic agent. It causes hypoglycemia by stimulating the release of insulin from the pancreas and increases peripheral sensitivity to insulin. The drug is well absorbed upon oral administration and is biotransformed by the liver. Its duration of action is about 12 to 24 h, whereas the duration of action of chlorpropamide is 1 to 3 days. Glyburide has a mild course of action, whereas chlorpropamide can cause water retention and dilutional hyponatremia. In addition chlorpropamide may decrease tolerance to ethanol in that ethanol in the presence of chlorpropamide causes flushing of the skin, particularly in the facial area. Glyburide has not been reported to cause this effect when ethanol is consumed.

**442. The answer is b.** (*DiPalma, 4/e, pp 458–462, 606–607. Hardman and Limbird, 9/e, pp 1468–1470.*) The concurrent administration of hydrocortisone and an oral hypoglycemic agent, such as chlorpropamide, reduces the effectiveness of the hypoglycemic agent in controlling blood glucose levels in patients who have noninsulin-dependent diabetes mellitus. Hydrocortisone and prednisone induce hyperglycemia by enhancing gluconeogenesis in the liver and periphery. In addition the steroids also promote the release of glucagon from the cells of the pancreas to eventually increase blood glucose levels. Hydrocortisone possesses significant mineralocorticoid activity in addition to its glucocorticoid effect. The mineralocorticoid action of hydrocortisone alters electrolyte metabolism. Hydrocortisone enhances the retention of Na and water in the body and augments the secretion of K, which can lead to hypokalemia. Prednisone also possesses a degree of mineralocorticoid activity and may produce hypokalemia. The diuretics hydrochlorothiazide and bumetanide can cause hypokalemia. In addition these diuretics cause hyperglycemia by inhibiting the release of insulin from the pancreas. If patients are to receive hydrocortisone and a loop or a thiazide diuretic, their K levels should be monitored to prevent K depletion.

**443. The answer is e.** (*DiPalma, 4/e, pp 586, 604, 607. Hardman and Limbird, 9/e, pp 1507–1509.*) Oral hypoglycemic agents are used in the treatment of patients with NIDDM. Chlorpropamide is a sulfonylurea compound that regulates blood glucose levels by promoting the secretion of insulin from β cells in the pancreas. Caution must be exercised when other drugs are given concomitantly with oral hypoglycemic agents. The effectiveness of chlorpropamide can be reduced by drugs such as phenobarbital, rifampin, thiazide and loop diuretics, phenytoin, and diazoxide. Phenobarbital and rifampin induce the biotransformation of oral hypoglycemic agents. The thiazides (e.g., chlorothiazide) and loop diuretic drugs (e.g., furosemide) as well as diazoxide reduce the hypoglycemic effect of chlorpropamide by inhibiting the secretion of insulin from the pancreas. Examples of some drugs that enhance the hypoglycemic action of chlorpropamide and other such compounds are aspirin, ethanol, $H_2$-receptor antagonists, probenecid, and sulfonamides.

**444–446. The answers are 444-a, 445-e, 446-d.** (*AMA Drug Evaluations Annual, 1993, pp 969, 971, 977, 1153, 2040. DiPalma, 4/e, pp 463, 624, 636–637, 644–645, 649.*) Mifepristone is structurally related to norethindrone. This compound is classified as a progesterone antagonist with weak agonistic properties. It can induce an abortion by causing contraction of the myometrium, which leads to detachment of the embryo. The drug is used in a single or multiple dose followed by the administration of a prostaglandin to cause the abortion. Mifepristone is well absorbed following oral administration. It is biotransformed to several active products. Most of the parent compound and its metabolites are excreted in the feces.

Fludrocortisone is a synthetic steroid compound that exhibits profound mineralocorticoid activity and some glucocorticoid activity. Electrolyte and water metabolisms are affected by the administration of this compound. Fludrocortisone promotes the reabsorption of Na and the urinary excretion of K and hydrogen ions in the collecting duct of the nephron. The drug is indicated for mineralocorticoid replacement therapy in primary adrenal insufficiency.

Leuprolide is a peptide that is related to GnRH or LHRH. This agent is used to treat metastatic prostate carcinoma. A hypogonadal state is produced in the patient from the continuous administration of leuprolide. Testosterone levels in the body become significantly reduced.

**447–449. The answers are 447-a, 448-b, 449-b.** (*DiPalma, 4/e, pp 584, 587–589. Hardman and Limbird, 9/e, pp 1397–1406.*) Agents that can interfere directly or indirectly with the synthesis of thyroid hormone are called *thyroid inhibitors.* Thiocyanate, an ionic inhibitor, interferes with the ability of the thyroid to concentrate $I^-$ by acting as a competitive inhibitor. Thiocyanate and other ionic inhibitors, such as perchlorate, nitrate, and fluoborate, are hydrated monovalent anions having a size similar to that of $I^-$.

Methimazole, together with PTU, is classified as an antithyroid drug that interferes directly with thyroid hormone synthesis. Antithyroid drugs interfere with the oxidation and incorporation of $I^-$ into organic form and inhibit the formation of iodothyronines from the peroxidase-mediated coupling of iodotyrosines. These drugs may act by binding to peroxidase, by interacting with substrates, or by interfering with the production of hydrogen peroxide, which (in addition to oxygen) is a biologic oxidant required for the synthesis of thyroid hormones.

$I^-$, most ancient of therapeutic agents for thyroid disorders, inhibits the secretion of thyroid hormone by retarding both the pinocytosis of colloid and proteolysis. This effect is observed in euthyroid as well as hyperthyroid persons.

Triiodothyronine is not classified as a thyroid inhibitor; it is an amino acid derivative of thyronine and results from the oxidative coupling of monoiodotyrosyl and diiodotyrosyl residues.

$^{131}I$, the most often used radioisotope of I, is rapidly absorbed by the thyroid and is deposited in follicular colloid. From the site of its deposition, $^{131}I$ causes fibrosis of the thyroid subsequent to pyknosis and necrosis of the follicular cells.

**450. The answer is b.** (*Hardman and Limbird, 9/e, p 1507. Katzung, 7/e, p 696.*) Three proposed mechanisms for sulfonylurea action are the release of insulin from pancreatic cells, reduction of serum glucagon levels, and increased binding of insulin to tissue receptors. On binding to a specific receptor associated with a K channel in cell membranes, sulfonylureas inhibit K efflux, which causes influx of Ca followed by release of preformed insulin.

**451. The answer is c.** *(Hardman and Limbird, 9/e, pp 1395–1396; Katzung, 7/e, p 629.)* The bound and the free concentration of $T_4$ will decrease unless this patient receives more drug. In a normal pregnant woman, the thyroid gland will secrete more $T_3$ and $T_4$ until the free levels are back in the normal range. However, after thyroidectomy or in any pregnant woman with hypothyroidism, exogenous thyroid hormone is required to maintain normal free levels. Also, the hypothyroid state must be corrected before administering oral contraceptives because they increase levels of thyroid-binding globulin.

**452. The answer is c.** *(Hardman and Limbird, 9/e, p 1401.)* PTU is more strongly protein bound and crosses the placenta to a lesser degree than methimazole and is therefore the safest antithyroid drug in pregnancy.

**453–455. The answers are 453-g, 454-e, 455-l.** *(AMA Drug Evaluations Annual, 1993, pp 1030–1031, 1137. DiPalma, 4/e, pp 463–464, 617, 627.)* Ethinyl estradiol is a synthetic estrogen derivative that is orally effective. It is used in combination with progestins as an oral contraceptive. Ethinyl estradiol is also used alone in various gynecologic disorders such as menopausal symptoms, breast cancer in selected postmenopausal women, and prostatic carcinoma. A major adverse reaction with ethinyl estradiol and other estrogens involves the coagulation reaction. Estrogens increase the synthesis of vitamin K-dependent factors II, VII, IX, and X. The effect on the coagulation scheme can alter the prothrombin time of persons who are using oral anticoagulants (e.g., warfarin). In addition, estrogens can increase the incidence of thromboembolic disorders through their procoagulation effect.

In the therapy of diabetes mellitus the effectiveness of insulin to regulate glucose levels in the body can be reduced by simultaneous administration of other drugs. Glucose levels in the body are elevated by the administration of glucocorticoid (e.g., hydrocortisone), dextrothyroxine, epinephrine, thiazide diuretics (e.g., hydrochlorothiazide), and $LT_4$. The drug-induced hyperglycemia counteracts the hypoglycemic action of insulin preparations. In addition, any drug that induces hyperglycemia can also reduce the effectiveness of the oral hypoglycemic agents such as tolbutamide, acetohexamide, and glyburide.

Spironolactone is classified as a K-sparing diuretic. Spironolactone is a competitive inhibitor of aldosterone. It has a mild diuretic effect but is generally used with other diuretics such as thiazides or loop diuretics to prevent the development of hypokalemia. The drug is also used in endocrinology in the diagnosis and treatment of hyperaldosteronism. Another therapeutic use of spironolactone is in the treatment of hirsutism in females, whether it is idiopathic or related to excessive androgen secretion. The drug causes a decrease in the rate of growth and the density of facial hair, possibly through inhibition of excessive androgen production and an effect on the hair follicle.

**456. The answer is e.** (*Hardman and Limbird, 9/e, p 1395.*) Thyroid hormone is used for hormone replacement therapy (HRT) in hypothyroidism. $T_4$ is the hormone of choice because of its consistent potency and prolonged duration of action.

**457. The answer is d.** (*Hardman and Limbird, 9/e, p 1481.*) Of the glucocorticoids listed, dexamethasone is the most potent. The dexamethasone suppression test has several uses—it not only allows complete suppression of pituitary ACTH production, but accurate measurement of endogenous corticosteroids as 17-ketosteroids in the urine. The small amount of dexamethasone present contributes minimally to this measurement.

**458. The answer is a.** (*Katzung, 7/e, p 643.*) Fetal lung maturation is normally stimulated by cortisol produced in the fetal adrenal gland. When preterm delivery with inadequate maturation of the lungs is anticipated, large doses of glucocorticoid can be given to the mother to speed up the physiologic process. Betamethasone is the preferred agent because it binds to serum proteins to a lesser extent than cortisol and other glucocorticoids, allowing more steroid to cross the placenta.

**459. The answer is a.** (*Hardman and Limbird, 9/e, pp 1482–1483. Katzung, 7/e, pp 647–648.*) Metyrapone inhibits 11-hydroxylation of steroid precursors, which prevents formation of cortisone and cortisol. These precursors are then diverted into aldosterone and androgen production pathways, which explains the adverse effects of hirsutism and edema.

**460. The answer is c.** (*Hardman and Limbird, 9/e, p 666.*) Inhalation therapy minimizes systemic effects. Of the agents above, beclomethasone is the only one delivered by metered-dose inhaler (MDI).

**461. The answer is b.** (*Hardman and Limbird, 9/e, p 1453. Katzung, 7/e, p 678.*) Finasteride is a competitive inhibitor of the steroid 5-reductase, causing reduction in plasma and prostate dihydrotestosterone. Males with benign prostatic hypertrophy (BPH) that are treated with finasteride are found to have decreased prostate size. A change in symptoms related to urination occurs in about one-third of patients.

**462. The answer is d.** (*Hardman and Limbird, 9/e, p 1401.*) In patients who are suspected of having hyperthyroidism, propranolol can be administered to provide temporary relief of the peripheral manifestations of the disease while the patient is further evaluated. Propranolol suppresses adrenergic symptoms such as tremors and tachycardia; it has no effect on the release of thyroid hormones from the gland.

*basic Point*

**463. The answer is g.** (*Hardman and Limbird, 9/e, p 1268.*) Plicamycin (mithramycin) can be used to treat hypercalcemia associated with malignancies. Its mechanism of action involves inhibition of Ca reabsorption from bone, leading to a reduction in serum Ca levels.

**464. The answer is e.** (*Hardman and Limbird, 9/e, p 1274.*) Medroxyprogesterone is used as a second-line hormone therapy for metastatic breast or endometrial carcinoma previously treated with surgery and radiation.

# TOXICOLOGY

Air Pollutants
  Benzene
  Carbon monoxide (CO)
  Carbon tetrachloride
  Chloroform
  Nitrogen dioxide ($NO_2$)
  Ozone
  Sulfur dioxide ($SO_2$)
  Tetrachloroethylene
  Toluene
  1,1,1–Trichloroethane
  Trichloroethylene
Alcohols
  Ethanol (ETH)
  Methanol
  Ethylene glycol
Heavy Metals
  Aluminum (Al)
  Arsenic (As)
  Cadmium (Cd)
  Gold (Au)

  Iron (Fe)
  Lead (Pb)
  Mercury (Hg)
  Zinc (Zn)
Heavy Metal Antagonists
  Edetate calcium disodium
    ($CaNa_2EDTA$)
  Deferoxamine
  Dimercaprol
  Penicillamine
Herbicide
  2,4-Dichlorophenoxyacetic acid
Organophosphorus Insecticides
  Diazinon
  Malathion
  Parathion
  Antidotes: atropine and
    pralidoxime
Toxic Gas
  Carbon monoxide (CO)
Toxic Ion

# Questions

**DIRECTIONS:** Each question below contains several suggested responses. Select the **one best** response to each question.

**465.** Convulsions caused by drug poisoning are most commonly associated with

a. phenobarbital
b. diazepam
c. strychnine
d. chlorpromazine
e. phenytoin

*(Inhibitory Neurons)*

**466.** Alkalinization of the urine with sodium bicarbonate is useful in the treatment of poisoning with

a. aspirin (acetylsalicylic acid)
b. amphetamine
c. morphine
d. phencyclidine
e. cocaine

**467.** Which of the following is an agent useful in the treatment of severe poisoning by organophosphorus insecticides, such as parathion?

a. ethylenediaminotetraacetic acid (EDTA)
b. pralidoxime (2-PAM)
c. N-acetylcysteine
d. carbachol
e. diethyldithiocarbamic acid

**468.** N-acetylbenzoquinoneimine is the hepatotoxic metabolite of which drug?

a. sulindac
b. acetaminophen (N-acetyl-para-aminophenol [APAP])
c. isoniazid (INH)
d. indomethacin
e. procainamide

**469.** Rapid intravenous (IV) administration of this drug causes hypocalcemic tetany

a. dimercaprol
b. edetate calcium disodium (Na$_2$ EDTA)
c. deferoxamine
d. penicillamine
e. N-acetylcysteine

**470.** Acute intermittent porphyria is a contraindication of the use of

a. enflurane
b. nitrous oxide (N$_2$O)
c. ketamine
d. diazepam
e. thiopental

**DIRECTIONS:** Each numbered question or incomplete statement below is NEGATIVELY phrased. Select the **one best** lettered response.

**471.** Characteristic features of arsenic poisoning include all the following EXCEPT

a. acute poisoning causes severe diarrhea and difficulty swallowing
b. signs of chronic poisoning include peripheral neuritis, hypotension, and anemia
c. death following acute intoxication may be due to hypovolemic shock
d. dimercaprol is the primary agent used in the treatment of chronic arsenic poisoning
e. gingivitis, stomatitis, and salivation can occur

**472.** Cadmium (Cd) poisoning is almost as common as Pb and Hg poisoning. Its features include all the following EXCEPT

a. it is commonly the main metal in certain types of batteries
b. exposure to fumes causes dyspnea, substernal discomfort, myalgias, headaches, and vomiting
c. chronic exposure results in severe liver injury
d. the most common long-term toxicity is renal
e. in Japan a Cd intoxication syndrome is known as *itai-itai* ("ouch-ouch") because of back, joint, and bone pain

**473.** Activated charcoal may be used to treat poisoning by all the following drugs EXCEPT

a. phenobarbital
b. carbamazepine
c. propoxyphene
d. lithium
e. aspirin

**474.** Methanol is a frequent cause of poisoning in alcoholics. Methanol intoxication differs from ethanol intoxication in all the following ways EXCEPT

a. blurred vision and hyperemia of the optic disc may develop
b. it may produce bradycardia, coma, and seizures
c. treatment includes administration of ethanol
d. ascorbic acid corrects the metabolic alkalosis
e. treatment may include hemodialysis

**475.** All the following drugs may produce a syndrome of flushing, headache, nausea, vomiting, sweating, hypotension, and confusion after ethanol consumption EXCEPT

a. amitriptyline
b. cefoperazone
c. acetohexamide
d. moxalactam
e. disulfiram

**476.** All the following statements are characteristic of carbon monoxide (CO) poisoning EXCEPT

a. poisoning is effectively treated with 100% oxygen ($O_2$)
b. it binds to hemoglobin (Hgb), reducing the $O_2$-carrying capacity of blood
c. carboxyhemoglobin (HbCO) levels below 15% rarely produce symptoms
d. symptoms of poisoning include headache, convulsions, and respiratory and cardiovascular depression
e. it inhibits ferricytochrome oxidase

**477.** Zinc (Zn) is an essential element for normal growth and development. However, toxicity can occur from excessive exposure. Manifestations of chronic poisoning include all the following EXCEPT

a. hyperamylasemia
b. thrombocytopenia
c. anemia
d. encephalopathy
e. fever

**DIRECTIONS:** Each group of questions below consists of lettered headings followed by a set of numbered items. For each numbered item select the **one** lettered heading with which it is **most** closely associated. Each lettered heading may be used **once, more than once, or not at all.**

### Questions 478–479

Many drugs when given to a pregnant woman produce significant adverse effects on the fetus. For each of the drugs below, match the most likely adverse effect.

a. vaginal adenocarcinoma
b. congenital goiter, hypothyroidism
c. masculinization of female fetus
d. "gray baby" syndrome
e. prolonged neonatal hypoglycemia
f. kernicterus

**478.** Testosterone

**479.** Methimazole

### Questions 480–481

For each patient, select the drug or agent most likely to cause the toxic effect.

a. aluminum (Al)
b. bismuth (Bi)
c. carbon monoxide (CO)
d. dapsone
e. methanol
f. gentamicin
g. lead (Pb)
h. metronidazole
i. nalidixic acid
j. primaquine
k. ethylene glycol
l. sulfamethoxazole
m. sulfasalazine
n. tetracycline

**480.** A 49-year-old woman is treated for an *Escherichia coli* urinary tract infection (UTI). During treatment the woman experiences hemolysis.

**481.** A three-year-old boy consumed a liquid from a container in the family garage. He shows central nervous system (CNS) depression, acidosis, suppressed respiration, and oxalate crystals in the urine. Beside supportive and corrective measures, ethanol was administered to the child.

### Questions 482–483

Certain drugs carry a risk of fetal abnormalities if administered during pregnancy. Match each abnormality with the correct drug.

a. penicillamine
b. diethylstilbestrol
c. prednisone
d. chloramphenicol
e. phenobarbital
f. disulfiram
g. ethanol
h. heroin
i. metronidazole
j. chlorambucil

**482.** Malformations of the genitourinary (GU) tract

**483.** Cutis laxa

## Questions 484–485

Death from acute poisoning usually occurs by mechanisms that involve vital systems such as respiration, circulation, or the CNS. Match each clinical picture with the causative agent.

a. cocaine
b. CO
c. strychnine
d. atropine
e. phenobarbital
f. heroin
g. phencyclidine
h. aspirin
i. cyanide
j. lysergic acid diethylamide (LSD)

*Atropine*

**484.** Hallucinations, delirium, and coma along with tachycardia and hypertension; hot, dry skin; urinary retention; and dilated pupils

**485.** Confusion, lethargy, and seizures; hyperventilation and hyperthermia; anion gap metabolic acidosis with dehydration and potassium (K) loss    *Aspirin*

# TOXICOLOGY

## Answers

**465. The answer is c.** (*Hardman and Limbird, 9/e, pp 89–90.*) Strychnine acts as a competitive antagonist of glycine, the predominant postsynaptic inhibitory transmitter in the brain and spinal cord. The fatal adult dose is 50 to 100 mg. Persons poisoned by strychnine suffer convulsions that progress to full tetanic convulsions. Because the diaphragm and thoracic muscles are fully contracted, the patient cannot breathe. Hypoxia eventually causes medullary paralysis and death. Control of the convulsions and respiratory support are the immediate objectives of therapy. Diazepam may be preferred to a barbiturate in controlling the convulsions because it offers less concomitant respiratory depression. Poisoning caused by the other drugs listed in the question is not associated with convulsions but with depression of the CNS.

**466. The answer is a.** (*DiPalma, 4/e, p 53. Hardman and Limbird, 9/e, pp 16–20.*) Sodium bicarbonate is excreted principally in the urine and alkalinizes it. Increasing urinary pH interferes with the passive renal tubular reabsorption of organic acids (such as aspirin and phenobarbital) by increasing the ionic form of the drug in the tubular filtrate. This would increase their excretion. Excretion of organic bases (such as amphetamine, cocaine, phencyclidine, and morphine) would be enhanced by acidifying the urine.

**467. The answer is b.** (*DiPalma, 4/e, pp 161–162, 259, 360. Hardman and Limbird, 9/e, p 170.*) The organophosphorus insecticides inactivate cholinesterases, which results in accumulation of endogenous acetylcholine in nerve tissue and effector organs. Very severe cases of acute poisoning should be treated first with atropine followed immediately by IV 2-PAM. Atropine inhibits the actions of acetylcholine at muscarinic cholinergic receptors, whereas 2-PAM reactivates the inactivated cholinesterases. The effectiveness of 2-PAM in reversing cholinesterase inhibition depends on early treatment inasmuch as the "aged" inhibited enzyme cannot be reactivated. Diethyldithiocarbamic acid is the active biotransformation product of disulfiram, which is an irreversible inhibitor of aldehyde dehydrogenase. N-acetylcysteine is an antidote used in the treatment of acetaminophen overdosage to prevent hepatotoxicities. Carbachol is a cholinomimetic drug and EDTA is a chelating agent. These compounds have no therapeutic value in the treatment of organophosphate poisoning.

**468. The answer is b.** (*DiPalma, 4/e, pp 357, 360, 413, 748. Hardman and Limbird, 9/e, pp 632–633.*) Hepatic necrosis can occur with overdosage of acetaminophen. The hepatic toxicity is the result of the biotransformation of acetaminophen to N-acetylbenzoquinoneimine, which reacts with hepatic proteins and glutathione. This metabolite depletes glutathione, stores and produces necrosis. The administration of N-acetylcysteine restores hepatic concentrations of glutathione and reduces the potential hepatotoxicity. Sulindac is biotransformed to sulindac sulfide, the active form of the drug. Both sulindac and its metabolites are excreted in the urine and in the feces. Indomethacin undergoes a demethylation reaction and an N-deacylation reaction. The parent compound and its metabolites are mainly excreted in the urine. Procainamide is converted to an active metabolite by an acetylation reaction. The product that is formed is N-acetylprocainamide (NAPA). In addition, procainamide is hydrolyzed by amidases. An N-acetylation reaction occurs also in the biotransformation of isoniazid. In the liver the enzyme N-acetyl transferase converts isoniazid to acetyl-isoniazid.

**469. The answer is b.** (*DiPalma, 4/e, pp 360, 509–510, 831–834. Hardman and Limbird, 9/e, pp 1664–1669.*) The chelation agent Na$_2$EDTA causes hypocalcemic tetany on rapid IV administration. This effect of Na$_2$EDTA is not observed on slow infusion (15 mg/min) since extracirculatory stores are available to prevent a significant reduction in plasma calcium levels. When CaNa$_2$EDTA is given IV, hypocalcemia does not develop even when large doses are required. CaNa$_2$EDTA is used in the diagnosis and treatment of Pb intoxication. Na$_2$EDTA is used to treat acute hypercalcemia. The other drugs listed do not cause hypocalcemia. Dimercaprol (British antilewisite [BAL]) forms chelation complexes between its sulfhydryl groups and metals and is used in the treatment of arsenic and Hg poisoning as well as in certain cases of Pb poisoning in children. Penicillamine is the drug of choice in treating Wilson's disease. The agent is also used in the therapy of copper, Hg, and Pb poisoning. N-acetylcysteine is an antidote used in the treatment of overdosage with acetaminophen to prevent hepatoxicity.

**470. The answer is e.** *(DiPalma, 4/e, p 239. Hardman and Limbird, 9/e, p 323.)* Induction of anesthesia by parenteral administration of thiopental sodium and other barbiturates is absolutely contraindicated in patients who have acute intermittent porphyria. These patients have a defect in regulation of δ-aminolevulinic acid synthetase; thus, administration of a barbiturate that increases this enzyme may cause a dangerous increase in levels of porphyrins. Administration of a barbiturate would exacerbate the symptoms of gastrointestinal and neurologic disturbances, cause extensive demyelination of peripheral and cranial nerves, and could lead to death.

**471. The answer is e.** *(DiPalma, 4/e, pp 826–827. Hardman and Limbird, 9/e, pp 1660–1661.)* Arsenic is an active constituent of fungicides, herbicides, and pesticides. Symptoms of acute toxicity include tightness in the throat, difficulty in swallowing, and stomach pains. Projectile vomiting and severe diarrhea can lead to hypovolemic shock and death. Chronic poisoning may cause peripheral neuritis, anemia, skin keratosis, and capillary dilation leading to hypotension. Dimercaprol is the primary agent used in the treatment of arsenic poisoning. Gingivitis, stomatitis, and salivation are symptoms associated with acute Hg poisoning.

**472. The answer is c.** *(DiPalma, 4/e, pp 829–830. Hardman and Limbird, 9/e, pp 1663–1664.)* The liver appears to be spared in cadmium intoxication. Not so the kidney, which in chronic exposure develops proteinuria with extensive damage to the proximal tubule. The symptoms of acute exposure to cadmium fumes are substernal discomfort, myalgias, headache, fatigue, and vomiting. These may be followed in severe cases by wheezing, hemoptysis, and pulmonary edema. In certain parts of Japan, where cadmium industrial waste is common, a syndrome of osteomalacia and bone deformities accompanied by pain and waddling gait is known as *itai-itai* (ouch-ouch).

**473. The answer is d.** *(DiPalma, 4/e, pp 288, 807. Hardman and Limbird, 9/e, p 72.)* Activated charcoal, a fine, black powder with a high adsorptive capacity, is considered to be a highly valuable agent in the treatment of many kinds of drug poisoning. Drugs that are well adsorbed by activated charcoal include primaquine, propoxyphene, dextroamphetamine, chlorpheniramine, phenobarbital, carbamazepine, digoxin, and aspirin. Mineral acids, alkalines, tolbutamide, and other drugs that are insoluble in acidic aqueous solution are not well adsorbed. Charcoal also does not bind cyanide, lithium, or iron.

**474. The answer is d.** (*DiPalma, 4/e, p 260. Hardman and Limbird, 9/e, p 1681–1682.*) Acute intoxication with methanol is common in chronic alcoholics. Headache, vertigo, vomiting, abdominal pain, dyspnea, blurred vision, and hyperemia of the optic disc can occur. Visual disturbances are caused by damage of retinal cells and the optic nerve by methanol metabolites. Severe cases of intoxication can lead to blindness. Other symptoms include bradycardia, prolonged coma, seizures, acidosis, and death by respiratory depression. Since methanol is biotransformed by alcohol dehydrogenase to highly toxic products (formaldehyde and formic acid), ethanol, which has high affinity for the enzyme, is useful in therapy because it reduces the biotransformation of methanol. Other treatments include hemodialysis to enhance removal of methanol and its products and alkalinization to reverse metabolic acidosis. 4-Methyl-prazole, an inhibitor of alcohol dehydrogenase, has also been proposed for treatment. Treatment with ascorbic acid would aggravate the acidosis.

**475. The answer is a.** (*DiPalma, 4/e, pp 259–260. Hardman and Limbird, 9/e, pp 391–392.*) Disulfiram is a pharmacologic adjunct in the treatment of alcoholism. When given to a person who has consumed ethanol, it produces flushing, headache, nausea, vomiting, sweating, hypotension, and confusion. The mechanism involves inhibition of aldehyde dehydrogenase; thus acetaldehyde accumulates as a result of ethanol metabolism. Many other agents produce disulfiram-like reactions when administered with ethanol, though their mechanisms have not been established; these include cephalosporins (cefoperazine, cefoperazone, moxalactam), phentolamine, metronidazole, and the sulfonylureas (e.g., acetohexamide and tolbutamide). The tricyclic antidepressant amitriptyline causes sedation. The interaction between ethanol and amitriptyline produces an enhancement of the central depressant properties of ethanol.

**476. The answer is e.** (*DiPalma, 4/e, pp 811–813. Hardman and Limbird, 9/e, pp 1676–1678.*) CO is a common cause of accidental and suicidal poisoning. Its affinity for hemoglobin is 250 times greater than that of $O_2$. It therefore binds to hemoglobin and reduces the $O_2$-carrying capacity of blood. The symptoms of poisoning are due to tissue hypoxia and progress from headache and fatigue to confusion, syncope, tachycardia, coma, convulsions, shock, respiratory depression, and cardiovascular collapse. Carboxyhemoglobin levels below 15% rarely produce symptoms; above 40%

symptoms become severe. Treatment includes establishment of an airway, supportive therapy, and administration of 100% $O_2$. It is the cyanide ion that binds to ferricytochrome oxidase and impairs cellular $O_2$ use, which leads to histotoxic hypoxia.

**477. The answer is d.** (*DiPalma, 4/e, pp 828–829.*) Unlike Pb, Hg, and Bi poisoning, chronic Zn poisoning does not manifest itself by CNS involvement. It can cause anemia and thrombocytopenia. Pancreatic involvement causes a decrease in secretion of amylase. Fever is a common symptom.

**478–479. The answers are 478-c, 479-b.** (*DiPalma, 4/e, pp 588, 606, 618, 742. Katzung, 7/e, p 979–982.*) There are many drugs that can produce significant adverse effects on the fetus when given to a pregnant woman. Among these are diethylstilbestrol, which has been shown to produce vaginal adenocarcinoma in female offspring. The incidence of clear-cell vaginal and cervical adenocarcinoma in women exposed to estrogens in utero has been estimated at 0.01% to 0.1%. Methimazole may cause hypothyroidism and congenital goiter by reducing thyroid hormone synthesis. Testosterone and derivatives can produce masculinization of the female fetus. Owing to low levels of glucuronyl transferase in the fetus, chloramphenicol increases the risk of "gray baby" syndrome. Sulfonylurea derivatives (e.g., chlorpropamide) can cause prolonged hypoglycemia in the neonate by stimulating excessive insulin secretion.

**480–481. The answers are 480-l, 481-k.** (*DiPalma, 4/e, pp 260–261, 738, 755, 779, 821–824. Hardman and Limbird, 9/e, pp 1061–1062, 1682–1683.*) Sulfonamides can cause acute hemolytic anemia. In some patients it may be related to a sensitization phenomenon and in other patients the hemolysis is due to a glucose-6-phosphate dehydrogenase deficiency. Sulfamethoxazole alone or in combination with trimethoprim is used to treat UTIs. The sulfonamide sulfasalazine is employed in the treatment of ulcerative colitis. Dapsone, a drug used in the treatment of leprosy, and primaquine, an antimalarial agent, can produce hemolysis, particularly in patients with a glucose-6-phosphate dehydrogenase deficiency.

Ethylene glycol, an industrial solvent and an antifreeze compound, is involved in accidental and intentional poisonings. This compound is initially oxidized by alcohol dehydrogenase and then further biotransformed to oxalic acid and other products. Oxalate crystals are found in various tissues of the body and are excreted by the kidney. Deposition of oxalate crystals in the kidney causes renal toxicity. Ethylene glycol is also a CNS depressant. In cases of ethylene glycol poisoning, ethanol is administered to reduce the first step in the biotransformation of ethylene glycol and, thereby, prevent the formation of oxalate and other products.

Pb poisoning in children is most often caused by the ingestion of paint chips that contain Pb. Older housing units and homes were painted with Pb compounds that produced various colors. Chronic Pb intoxication causes such symptoms as basophilic stippling, increased δ-aminolevulinic aciduria, tremors, weakness of extensor muscles, constipation, lead line, and colic.

**482–483. The answers are 482-j, 483-a.** *(Katzung, 7/e, p 983.)* Practically every drug has warnings concerning administration during pregnancy. Most warn of the increased risk of deformities of limb development and defects like cleft palate. A few drugs carry the risk of distinct organ defects. For example, chlorambucil may cause agenesis of the fetal kidneys. Penicillamine seems to affect fetal connective tissue, causing relaxation of the skin, hypotonia, and hyperflexion of the hips and shoulders.

**484–485. The answers are 484-d, 485-h.** *(DiPalma, 4/e, pp 166–167, 352–353. Katzung, 7/e, p 972.)* Atropine blocks muscarinic cholinergic transmission in the brain and in the autonomic nervous system. The result is dry mouth, thirst, dry and hot skin, tachycardia, urinary retention, ataxia, restlessness, excitement, and hallucinations followed by stupor, delirium, respiratory depression, coma, and death.

Salicylate or aspirin overdose is characterized by tinnitus, confusion, rapid pulse rate, and increased respiration. The decreased partial pressure of arterial $CO_2$ ($PCO_2$) plus increased fixed acids at first cause alkalosis which is followed by metabolic acidosis and dehydration and loss of fixed bases. The picture may resemble diabetic acidosis, but the history of salicylate ingestion and blood salicylate levels above 540 mg/100 mL clinch the diagnosis.

# HIGH-YIELD FACTS

# HIGH-YIELD FACTS
## SAMPLE DRUG
## CLASSIFICATION TABLES

### TIPS FOR LEARNING PHARMACOLOGY

Pharmacology is best learned by comparing drugs within a particular class or by their specific use.

A chart highlighting the similarities and differences among the various agents can be a helpful tool. The charts included in this section are simple examples. More elaborate charts can be constructed that would include how the drug is administered, its pharmacological effects, its adverse effects, its mechanism of toxicity (if known), and significant drug-drug interactions. For infectious disease agents, the spectrum of antimicrobial activity and the basis of antibiotic resistance can be added.

Explanations for the abbreviations used in these charts are found in the List of Abbreviations and Acronyms, which appears before the Bibliography.

*Arnold Stern, M.D., Ph.D.*
*Professor of Pharmacology*
*New York University Medical Center*
*New York, NY*

## DRUGS FOR TREATING HYPERTENSION

| DRUG CLASS | PROTOTYPE | ACTION |
|---|---|---|
| **Sympathetic Nervous System Agents** | | |
| Central | clonidine | $\alpha_2$-agonist; causes decreased sympathetic outflow |
| Peripheral | guanethidine | uptake by transmitter vesicles in nerve depletes and replaces norepinephrine in neurosecretory vesicles |
| | prazocin | $\alpha_1$-antagonist |
| | propranolol | $\beta$-antagonist |
| Central and Peripheral | reserpine | binds tightly to storage vesicles, which consequently lose their ability to concentrate and store norepinephrine |
| **Vasodilators** | | |
| Arterial | hydralazine | unknown |
| | diazoxide | opens $K^+$ channels and causes hyperpolarization of smooth muscle |
| Arterial and Venous | nitroprusside | releases NO, which binds to guanylyl cyclase to generate cGMP |
| **$Ca^{++}$ Channel-Blockers** | nifedipine | inhibits voltage-dependent "L-type" $Ca^{++}$ channels |
| **ACE Inhibitors** | captopril | inhibits conversion of angiotensin I to angiotensin II |
| **Diuretics** | | |
| Thiazides (Benzothiadiazides) | hydrochlorothiazide | inhibits $Na^+$ channels in luminal membrane in the proximal segment of the distal tubule |
| Loop Agents | furosemide | inhibits cotransporter of $Na^+$, $K^+$, $Cl^-$ in the ascending limb of the loop of Henle |

## DRUGS FOR TREATING BACTERIAL INFECTIOUS DISEASES

| DRUG CLASS | PROTOTYPE | ACTION | SPECTRUM |
|---|---|---|---|
| **Penicillins** | | inhibit bacterial cell wall synthesis by binding to penicillin-binding proteins, inhibiting cross-linking enzymes and activating autolytic enzymes that disrupt bacterial cell walls | streptococci, menigococci, pneumococci, Gram-positive bacilli, gonococci, spirochetes |
| Narrow Spectrum | | | |
| Penicillinase-susceptible | penicillin G | | |
| Penicllinase-resistant | methicillin | | staphylococci |
| Wide Spectrum Penicillinase-susceptible | ampicillin | | similar to penicillin G; also includes *E. coli, P. mirabilis*, and *H. influenzae* |
| | carbenicillin | | Gram-negative rods and especially useful for Pseudomonas species |
| **Cephalosporins** | | | |
| First-Generation | cephalothin | | Gram-positive cocci, *E. coli*, and *K. pneumoniae* |
| Second-Generation | cefamandole | | greater activity against Gram-negative organisms than first-generation cephalosporins |
| Third-Generation | cefoperazone | | broader activity against resistant Gram-negative organisms; some derivatives penetrate the blood brain-barrier |
| **Carbapenem** | imipenem | | wide action against Gram-positive cocci, Gram-negative rods, and some anaerobes |
| **Monobactam** | aztreonam | | resistant to $\beta$-lactamases produced by Gram-negative rods |
| **Macrolides** | erythromycin | inhibits protein synthesis by binding to part of the 50S ribosomal subunit | Gram-positive cocci, mycoplasma, corynebacteria, *Legionella, Ureaplasma, Bordetella* |

## DRUGS FOR TREATING BACTERIAL INFECTIOUS DISEASES (continued)

| DRUG CLASS | PROTOTYPE | ACTION | SPECTRUM |
|---|---|---|---|
| Vancomycin | vancomycin | inhibits synthesis of cell wall mucopeptides (peptidoglycans) | Gram-positive bacteria, especially for resistant mutants |
| Chloramphenicol | chloramphenicol | inhibits peptide bond formation by binding to the 50S ribosomal subunit, inhibiting peptidyl transferase | *Salmonella* and *Haemophilus* infections and meningococcal and pneumococcal meningitis |
| **Aminoglycosides** Systemic | gentamicin | inhibits protein synthesis by binding to the 30S subunit of ribosomes, which blocks formation of the initiation complex, causing misreading of the code on the mRNA template and disrupting polysomes | *E. coli, Enterobacter, Klebsiella, Proteus, Pseudomonas,* and *Serratia* species |
| Local | neomycin | | |
| Tetracycline | tetracycline | inhibits protein synthesis by binding to the 30S ribosomal subunit, which interferes with binding of aminoacyl-tRNA | mycoplasma, chlamydia, rickettsia, vibrio |
| Sulfa Drugs | sulfonamides | inhibit folic acid synthesis by competitive inhibition of dihydropteroate synthase | Gram-positive and -negative organisms, including chlamydia and nocardia |
| Trimethoprim | trimethoprim | inhibits folic acid synthesis by inhibition of dihydrofolate reductase | used in combination with sulfamethoxazole |
| Fluoroquinolones | norfloxacin | inhibits topoisomerase II (DNA gyrase) | Gram-negative organisms, including gonococci, *E. coli, K. pneumoniae, C. jejuni, Enterobacter, Salmonella,* and *Shigella* species |

# LIST OF ABBREVIATIONS AND ACRONYMS

α—alpha

*A. lumbricoides—Ascaris lumbricoides*

ABVD—adriamycin, bleomycin, vinblastine, and decarbazine

ACE inhibitor—angiotensin-converting enzyme inhibitor

acetyl-CoA—acetyl coenzyme A

ACH/Ach—acetylcholine

AchE—acetylcholinesterase

ACTH—adrenocorticotropic hormone

ADD—attention-deficit disorder

ADH—antidiuretic hormone (vasopressin [VP])

ADHD—attention deficit hyperactivity disorder

ADP—adenosine 5'-diphosphate

AF—atrial fibrillation

AHD—arteriosclerotic heart disease

AIDS—acquired immunodeficiency syndrome

Al—aluminum

$Al(OH)_3$—aluminum hydroxide

ALG—antilymphocyte globulin

AMP—adenosine monophosphate

ANS—autonomic nervous system

APAP—acetaminophen (*N*-acetyl-para-aminophenol)

As—arsenic

aspirin—acetylsalicylic acid

ATP—adenosine triphosphate

ATPase—adenosine triphosphatase

Au—gold

AUC—area under the (blood concentration-time) curve

AV—atrioventricular

$\beta$—beta

*B. fragilis—Bacteroides fragilis*

BAL—British antilewisite (dimercaprol)

BCG vaccine—Bacille bilié de Calmette-Guérin vaccine

Bi—bismuth

BPH—benign prostatic hypertrophy

BPM—breaths per minute; beats per minute

BUN—blood urea nitrogen


C—mean plasma concentration

$C_{max}$—maximum plasma concentration

$C_{min}$—minimum plasma concentration

*C. albicans—Candida albicans*

*C. botulinum—Clostridium botulinum*

*C. difficile—Clostridium difficile*

*C. jejuni—Campylobacter jejuni*

*C. neoformans—Cryptococcus neoformans*

Ca—calcium

$Ca^{++}$—calcium divalent cation

CaG—calcium gluconate

cAMP—adenosine 3',5'-cyclic monophosphate (cyclic AMP)

$CaNa_2EDTA$— edetate calcium disodium

CCNS—cell cycle—nonspecific

CCS—cell cycle—specific

Cd—cadmium

CD—cluster of differentiation

cGMP—guanosine 3'5'-cyclic monophosphate (cyclic GMP)

CHF—congestive heart failure

CK—creatine kinase

Cl—chlorine

$Cl^-$—chloride

$CL_{total}$—total body clearance

cm—centimeter

Cn—cyanide

CNS— central nervous system

CO—carbon monoxide

$CO_2$—carbon dioxide

COMT—catechol-$O$-methyltransferase
COPD—chronic obstructive pulmonary disease
corticotropin—adrenocorticotropic hormone (ACTH)
CRF—corticotropin releasing factor
CSF—cerebrospinal fluid

$\delta$—delta
$D_2$—dopamine receptor
*D. latum*—*Diphyllobothrium latum*
DHT—dihydrotestosterone
DM—dopamine (3,4-dihydroxyphenylethylamine)
DMMS—drug-metabolizing microsomal system
DNA—deoxyribonucleic acid
dopa/DOPA/Dopa—(3,4-dihydroxyphenylalanine)
DTIC—dacarbazine
DVT-deep—vein (venous) thrombosis

*E. coli*—*Escherichia coli*
*E. vermicularis*—*Enterobius vermicularis*
ED—emergency department
EDRF—endothelial-derived relaxing factor
EDTA—ethylenediaminetetraacetic acid
EEG—electroencephalogram
EGF—erythrocyte growth factor
EKG—electrocardiogram
ER—endoplasmic reticulum
ETH—ethanol

5-FU—5-fluorouracil
5-HT—5-hydroxytryptamine (serotonin)
$5\text{-HT}_{1D}$ receptors—5-hydroxytryptamine receptors (a subclass of
    serotonergic receptors)
15-methyl-$PGF_{2\alpha}$—15-methyl-prostaglandin $F_{2\alpha}$ (carboprost)
*F. hepatica*—*Fasciola hepatica*
FDA—Food and Drug Administration
Fe—iron
$FH_2$—7,8-dihydrofolic acid

$FH_4$—5,6,7,8-tetrahydrofolic acid
FSH—follicle-stimulating hormone
FU—fluorouracil

γ—gamma
G. lamblia—Giardia lamblia
G protein—guanine nucleotide-binding protein
GABA—γ-aminobutyric acid
G-CSF—granulocyte colony stimulating factor
GDP-GTP—guanine diphosphate and triphosphate
GERD—gastroesophageal reflux disease
GI—gastrointestinal
GM-CSF—granulocyte macrophage colony stimulating factor
GMP—guanylic acid
GnRH—gonadotropin-releasing hormone
GTP—guanosine triphosphate
GU—genitourinary

h—hour(s)
$H_2$—histamine$_2$
H. influenzae—Haemophilus influenzae
H. pylori—Helicobacter pylori
HbCO—carboxyhemoglobin
hCG—human chorionic gonadotropin
HCl—hydrochloride
HDL—high-density lipoprotein
Hg—mercury
Hgb—hemoglobin
HIV—human immunodeficiency virus
$H^+/K^+$/ATPase—hydrogen-potassium-adenosine triphosphatase
hMG—human menopausal gonadotropin
HMG—CoA-β-hydroxy-β-methylglutaryl-coenzyme A
HRT—hormone replacement therapy

IDDM—insulin-dependent diabetes mellitus
IgE, G—immunoglobulin E, G
IL-1, −2—interleukin-1, −2
IM—intramuscular(ly)

IND—investigational new drug (application)
INH—isoniazid
IP—interphalangeal/intraperitoneal(ly)
$IP_3$—inositol-1,4,5-trisphosphate
IRB—institutional review board
IV—intravenous(ly)

κ—kappa
$K^+$—potassium, univalent form
$k_e$—elimination rate constant
K. mobilis—Klebsiella mobilis
K. pneumoniae—Klebsiella pneumoniae
$KClO_4$—potassium perchlorate
kg—kilogram
KI—potassium iodide

L—liter
L/h—liters per hour
L. pneumophilia—Legionella pneumophilia
L-dopa—levodopa
L-thyroxine $(T_4)$—levothyroxine
"L-type" $Ca^{++}$ channels—L-type calcium channels (in muscles and
    neurons; have long, large, high thresholds of Ca current)
LDL—low-density lipoprotein
LHRH—luteinizing hormone-releasing hormone (hypothalamic)
LSD—lysergic acid diethylamide
LT—leukotriene

μ—mu
μg/mg—micrograms per milligram
μg/mL—micrograms per milliliter
MAO—monoamine oxidase
MAO-A, B—MAO type A, B
MAOI—monoamine oxidase inhibitor
MDI—metered-dose inhaler
mEq/L—milliequivalents per liter
mg—milligram
mg/min—milligrams per minute

Mg—magnesium
$Mg^{++}$—magnesium divalent cation
MI—myocardial infarction
MIF—migration inhibitory factor
min—minute(s)
mL/min—milliliters per minute
mmHg—millimeters of mercury
mRNA—messenger ribonucleic acid


N—nitrogen
$N_M$ receptors—nicotinic-muscular receptors found in skeletal muscle
   neuromuscular endplates
$N_N$ receptors—nicotinic-neural receptors found in parasympathetic
   ganglia
*N. americanus—Necator americanus*
*N. gonorrhoeae—Neisseria gonorrhoeae*
NA—nicotinic acid (niacin)
$Na^+$—sodium, univalent form
NaCl—sodium chloride
NADH—nicotinamide adenine dinucleotide
NADPH—nicotinamide adenine dinucleotide phosphate
$Na_2EDTA$—edetate disodium
NaI—sodium iodide
$Na^+/K^+/ATPase$—sodium-potassium-adenosine triphosphatase
$Na^+/K^+/2Cl^-$—sodium-potassium-dichloride
NAPA—*N*-acetylprocainamide
NDA—new drug application
NE—norepinephrine
ng/mL—nanograms per milliliter
NIDDM—noninsulin-dependent diabetes mellitus
NMDA—*N*-methyl-D-aspartate antagonists (glutamate channel)
NMN—normetanephrine
NMS—neuroleptic malignant syndrome
NO—nitric oxide
$N_2O$—nitrous oxide
$NO_2$—nitrogen dioxide
NPH—isophane
NPY—neuropeptide Y

NRC—National Research Council
NSAID—nonsteroidal anti-inflammatory drug (nonopioid analgesic)

$O_2$—oxygen

P—phosphorous
*P. aeruginosa—Pseudomonas aeruginosa*
*P. carinii—Pneumocystis carinii*
*P. kellicotti—Paragonimus kellicotti*
*P. mirabilis—Proteus mirabilis*
*P. vivax—Plasmodium vivax*
PABA—*p*-aminobenzoic acid
PAS—para-aminosalicylic acid
Pb—lead
PBP—penicillin-binding protein
$P_{CO_2}$—partial pressure (tension) of carbon dioxide, artery
PDGF—platelet-derived growth factor
$PGE_1$—prostaglandin $E_1$ (alprostadil)
$PGE_2$—prostaglandin $E_2$ (dinoprostone)
$PGI_2$—prostaglandin $I_2$ (prostacyclin)
PNS—peripheral nervous system
$P_{O_2}$—partial pressure (tension) of oxygen, arterial
PPD—purified protein derivative of tuberculin
protein G—guanine nucleotide-binding protein
PTH—parathyroid hormone
PTU—propylthiouracil
PVC—premature ventricular contraction

RDA—recommended daily allowance
REM—rapid eye movement
RNA—ribonucleic acid

6-MP—mercaptopurine
S—sulfur
*S. aureus— Staphylococcus aureus*
*S. haematobium—Schistosoma haematobium*
SA—sinoatrial
SAR—structure-activity relationship

SC—subcutaneous
sec—second(s)
SH—sulfhydryl
SL—sublingual
$SO_2$—sulfur dioxide
SRS-A—slow-reacting substance of anaphylaxis
SSRI—selective serotonin reuptake inhibitor
SVT—supraventricular tachycardia

2-PAM—pralidoxime
2-PAM Cl—pralidoxime chloride
$T_3$—triiodothyronine
$T_4$—thyroxine
*T. saginata—Taenia saginata*
tacrine—tetrahydroaminoacridine
TB—tuberculosis
thiazides—benzothiadiazides
TIA—transient ischemic attack
TNF—tumor necrosis factor
tPA—tissue plasminogen activator
TRH—thyroid/thyrotropin-releasing hormone
tRNA—transfer ribonucleic acid

USAN Council—United States Adopted Names Council
USMLE—United States Medical Licensing Examination
UTI—urinary tract infection

$V_d$—volume of distribution
VIP—vasoactive intestinal peptide
vitamin $B_1$—thiamine
vitamin $B_2$—riboflavin
vitamin $B_6$—pyridoxine
vitamin C—ascorbic acid
vitamin D—calcitriol (metabolite [active form-1,25-$(OH)_2D_3$])
VLDL—very-low-density lipoprotein
VP—vasopressin (antidiuretic hormone [ADH])
VT—ventricular tachycardia

*W. bancrofti—Wuchereria bancrofti*

Zn—zinc

# BIBLIOGRAPHY

*AMA Drug Evaluations Annual, 1993.* Chicago, American Medical Association, 1994

DiPalma JR, DiGregorio GJ, Barbieri EJ, Ferko AP: *Basic Pharmacology in Medicine, 4/e.* West Chester, PA, Medical Surveillance, 1994.

Hardman JG, Limbird LE (eds): *Goodman & Gilman's the Pharmacological Basis of Therapeutics, 9/e.* New York, McGraw-Hill, 1996.

Isselbacher KJ, et al (eds): *Harrison's Principles of Internal Medicine, 13/e.* New York, McGraw-Hill, 1994.

Katzung BG: *Basic and Clinical Pharmacology, 7/e.* East Norwalk, CT, Appleton & Lange, 1997.